From Couch To Life!

From Couch To Life!

YOUR HOW-TO MANUAL FOR PROFOUND HEALTH, HEALING AND BOUNDLESS ENERGY

Sue Lyndes

From Couch To Life!

sue@fromcouchtolife.com

The content of this book is for general instruction only. Each person's physical, emotional, and spiritual condition is unique. The instruction in this book is not intended to replace or interrupt the reader's relationship with a physician or other professional. Please consult your doctor for matters pertaining to your specific health and diet.

For more information, visit
www.fromcouchtolife.com

ISBN: 0692432108
ISBN 13: 9780692432105
Library of Congress Control Number: 2015909348
From Couch To Life!, Bishop, CA
Printed in the United States of America

Dedicated to my husband, Ken
who stayed with me even
when I wanted to leave myself.
Without his love, care and support,
I could not have completed this journey.
Thank you with all my heart!

Table of Contents

Acknowledgments

My mum and dad, for teaching me there's no such word as can't, that where there's a will, there's a way and that I can do anything I set my mind to. Though I may have sworn at you once or twice on my journey as I heard you repeat those words endlessly in my head, your belief in me gave me the courage to move forward. Though you are no longer with us, I felt you with me every step of the way.

The members of the Rotary Club of Bishop, whose fellowship and support have been instrumental in my recovery. You showed me how to have fun and live again! As a thank you to every one of you, I am donating 10% of each book sale to Rotary International. I am so proud to be a Rotarian!

Dr. Murat Akalin, for his skillful practice of treating me as a whole human being and helping to show me the way. Thank you for saving me from all those rabbit holes!

Foreword

"It is the greatest of all mistakes to do nothing because you can only do a little."

Sydney Smith

Introduction

Why *"From Couch to Life!"*

I called my book "From Couch To Life!" because that's what I did.

Sick for more than a decade, housebound for almost three years and receiving other people's immune systems in costly and lengthy monthly infusions in order to function, I didn't think it could get any worse. Then I started to develop an allergic reaction to my treatments. At that point, I thought it was the end of any kind of meaningful life for me.

As my health declined, my life and world got ever smaller until it was so tiny; I questioned the purpose of such an existence.

A closet writer all my life, in 2010, one of the only things I could find that I had written was on a post it note; *"The day passes in a haze of pain and despair."* Reading that even now, almost five years later, instantly brings a prick of tears to my eyes.

I spent hours sitting on the back deck of my home, looking up at the Sierra Nevada mountains, thinking that I would never get the chance to explore them. I wondered how it was possible to be so sick and yet have no answers, much less solutions.

Down to less than 100lbs in weight, eating was more exhausting than not eating and days would go by without any food passing my lips. The longer I went, the better I felt, until the lightheadedness, dizziness and exhaustion would force me to eat and the cycle of sickness would begin.

In hindsight, it's so obvious that the answer was right in front of me all along. Though there were some big clues, somehow I didn't put them together for a long, long time. It was the food I was eating that was making me so sick. Well, that and my reactions to all the things that had happened during my 53 years on this earth. Hindsight showed me how my diet and lifestyle choices had combined to put me precisely where I was.

For the first time, I really "got" the Mind/Body Connection and was awed by the intricate balance between all the aspects of our lives, though we barely concentrate on the basics.

So what exactly did I do to get myself from the couch to living a full, vibrant life as a health and wellness coach, published author and President of the Rotary Club of Bishop, all within five years?

Though you have heard it a million times before, there really is a way and the answer is easier than you think. Lack of information has never been the problem; how to take that information and make meaningful, long lasting change in our lives is the real challenge. In the great paradox of modern life where all information is instantly available, the more we read the more difficult it is to take action.

From Couch to Life!, takes you through an easy, Ten Step process, implementing small changes until before you know it, you are on the path to wellness in every area of your life. And you know what's best of all? **You** will have done this and discovered your wellness is not dependent on another human being, drug, the latest research, fad or doctor. You. Just you.

Let that sink in for a minute.

You'll be able to take control of your life, without the need for anything else. Once you know how the process works you'll be able to use it time and time again to work through all that life brings, allowing you to overcome obstacles and take advantage of opportunities.

How awesome is that?

As we go through these ten steps, I share my journey with you so you can see how I applied the principles to my own life and specific health challenges. It's important that you see I'm not some superhuman with extraordinary powers. No. I am just like you.

Having given up and found myself still frustratingly here on this earth, I decided against all odds and medical advice to find a way to pull myself off the couch and into a vibrant, action packed, blessed life that I couldn't even have imagined before I became sick. Bless my parents for instilling that indomitable spirit in me!

I still pinch myself when I look at all I get to do in a day and how far I've come by refusing to give in. In my lowest of times, when I thought I had given up, I was always aware of a tiny, tiny speck of light, hidden deep, deep inside me that refused to be extinguished.

The utter frustration and anger at being forced to wake up each morning to live such a life seemed to suck what little energy I had left right out of me, but, that little flame kept burning away, somehow defying the gale force winds trying to extinguish it. Just as my body, malnourished, skeletal, broken and in pain, somehow functioned day after day without fuel. My spirit remained broken but unbowed even in the face of utter defeat.

I'm describing my absolute bottom. I had nowhere to go. Having thrown in the towel, I was seriously ticked that I still had to drag myself through day after miserable day. After much swearing, temper tantrums and good old "poor me", victim reveling, I started to hear the clear, familiar words of my childhood, "You'll just have to make the most of what you have."

CHAPTER 1

Starting Your Journey

The Meaning of Life

The first step in my recovery was to figure out what the purpose of such a life was. If this is what I have to work with, I reasoned, I'd have to figure out a way to make life meaningful. I was hardly the first person in the world to have faced such challenges. Life is full of examples of how others have persevered against all odds to overcome seemingly insurmountable obstacles. I knew one thing for sure; if recovery was possible for one person, it was possible for me.

Here is part of an essay I wrote in 2008 as I struggled to process my thoughts and feelings.

The Purpose of Life

What is our purpose in life?

Chronically ill for many years, this is a question I have found myself returning to time and time again.

Having been unable to work for many years, I am aware that my life and purpose look very different to most people. As an example, the purpose of many lives seems to be to work, make a contribution, to be able to buy things we feel make our lives somehow happier and more fulfilled.

What is the purpose of someone who cannot participate in the mainstream ideals we are fed incessantly? Having been in that category for many years now, I have had to redefine and rethink my purpose.

I can't help but think "purpose" can't ever be about "doing", however that might look. After all, if it were about doing, then anyone who was unable to "do" would not have any purpose, which can't be right.

And what of all those "things" we accumulate throughout our lives that we think define our purpose? We sure as heck can't take it with us when we leave this current experience.

What of people who are paralyzed and unable to "do" anything? Does that mean they have no purpose? That I can't believe.

And who says there has to be a purpose anyway?

If there is a purpose to life, it's surely in the life itself; to be; to exist. Just because humans have the ability to ask the 'big questions" in life, such as who are we; where do we come from and what is our life purpose; does not mean there has to be a purpose attached to the ability.

So if purpose doesn't come from doing, what does it come from?

It seems to me the only thing that makes sense is to be. The only "doing" required is not one of physical but mental action. An expanded consciousness or idea about who we are in this world and the part we have to play in it."

I understood that if all I had to work with were my thoughts, I could at least make sure I contributed to the good thoughts of the world. The idea made me realize what it means to be a human "being," and became my driving force and the key that unlocked the door of my journey to health.

I realized if everyone had the luxury of time to contemplate such things and make a conscious effort to focus on the good, rather than the bad in life, we really would all live in the kind of world we all say we want to live in. Just like that, I had a purpose and what a purpose it was!

I went from feeling like a bump on the log of life as my life passed by at lightening speed, to having not just a purpose, but perhaps one of the most important I could have conceived. Contributing to the positive, healing thoughts of my community and world. The little spark grew almost imperceptibly brighter and so began my long journey to health and healing.

Did you notice that the first step on the road to wellness was not body, but mind and soul food?

Having figured out that I did have a life purpose and it was worth sticking around after all, my next step was to work out how to move forward.

Since becoming sick in December 2001, I have seen dozens of doctors, taken dozens of drugs and been subjected to medical procedures I didn't even know existed, all in my pursuit of answers and the ever elusive cure.

I've had endoscopies, colonoscopies, biopsies and been shot full of nuclear medicine. I have done so many blood tests; I could stock the national blood bank for years. I've had MRI's, CT scans, had ultrasound performed from tip to toe and tumors removed, benign thank goodness.

I wore a heart monitor for a month, was made to drink bicarbonate of soda while strapped upside down in a machine and now know why babies scream when they have colic. They gave me digestive enzymes, shut off my stomach pumps and finally, started infusing other people's immune systems into me. That last one worked, at least for nine glorious months when I was able to leave the couch and start enjoying life again.

I camped in the mountains, was able to drive again and even ventured to San Francisco some six hours away. Though the treatments made me sick for about a week, being able to live life again was like winning the lottery, though it came with a hefty price tag. The expense of the treatments decimated our bank account and made winning the lottery seem like the only solution to keep going.

I'm sure many reading this have similar stories.

Then the allergic reactions started and after changing medication several times, it became obvious my body was rejecting the treatment. It was, after all, a product made from the immune systems of hundreds of people.

Making the decision to stop was very hard.

My specialist had obtained authorization from my insurance company for a different kind of treatment, but I knew in my heart it wasn't the answer. I was so scared, walking away, knowing I was leaving the only shred of an answer behind. Life looked very small and dark again and I shuddered at what the future would bring.

I had no idea what was wrong with me, any more than the dozens of doctors I had seen did. One thing kept coming to my mind. Perhaps it was the change in my condition with the infusion treatments, but I was struck by the fact that when my body had what it needed, it functioned really well.

For some reason, beginning in 2001, ill health had become the default for my body and it kept replicating the same thing over and over in an endless cycle.

What if I gave my body a new blueprint for health?

I knew that on a cellular level, every part of the body is replaced over certain time periods. If I could just give it a different blueprint to work from, I might produce good health just as easily, given the right conditions.

> *"People may think of their body as a fairly permanent structure, most of it is in a state of constant flux as old cells are discarded and new ones generated in their place. Each kind of tissue has its own turnover time, depending in part on the workload endured by its cells. The cells lining the stomach, as mentioned, last only five days. The red blood cells, bruised and battered after traveling nearly 1,000 miles through the maze of the body's circulatory system, last only 120 days or so on average before being dispatched to their graveyard in the spleen."*

> Nicolas Wade, long time Science Writer, NY Times
> (*Reference: Dr. Frisen, Stem Cell Biologist, the Karolinska Institute, Stockholm, Sweden*)

Great plan, but how?

Believe Recovery Is Possible

Believing that recovery was possible was the first step in this process. If I believed an answer or cure was not possible, that it lay in the hands of someone else or that it only existed in the future, I would remain sick. This is one of the many ways body and mind are connected, but we'll get to that in more detail in Chapter Seven when we look at how food for the body and food for the mind and soul integrate.

Despite what it seems given that no one on the planet knows what is wrong with you, recovery is not only possible but absolutely can and will happen to you.

That's because there is a person who knows, and you don't even have to leave the house to see them. Just pick yourself off your couch as best you can at this stage in your journey and look in the mirror. You, yes you, are going to find not *THE* answer, but *YOUR* answer to getting your life back on track.

In the following Chapters, we are going to take a brief look at chronic disease in the United States and some of the more obvious reasons for it. Next, we'll delve into "Your Prescription for Health", and how you can begin your own journey to the life you know you are supposed to be living.

It all starts with this first crucial step; knowing that recovery IS possible and that you have all you need to get started on your own journey to health in all areas of your life.

Playing Your Way

As frustrating as it is, being stuck on the couch is what you have to contend with for now, but now you know you have reason and purpose and have started to understand recovery is possible. Your journey to health has begun.

In fact, taking the time to look at where you are and how you could make just one change – in your belief that recovery *is* possible – means you have already taken the first crucial step. Without that first step, no change is possible so congratulations, you are on your way. See how easy that was and how different life already looks, knowing recovery is within your grasp?

Is that the stirrings of hope in your heart as you dare to contemplate a life of doing as well as being, perhaps even fulfillment?

Back when I was looking for answers, I would come across so many well-meaning people who would tell me all kinds of unhelpful things. I'm sure we could all fill a book with the completely useless and soul-destroying things others have said to us in an attempt to help.

Trying to completely avoid the subject of religion and beliefs while talking about it openly, many of the comments I found hard to stomach were in the vein that my belief in God was somehow deficient. If only I would give myself completely, salvation and healing were to be mine. I tried to understand what they were saying, but it took months to see the bright side of these insulting comments!

What struck me about this approach was the assumption there was something wrong with me in the first place. Yes, I know, this is a book about my rise from disease-ridden couch to life, so clearly, there was a lot wrong!

Perhaps, on the outside that was true. I could not deny my body was broken, my spirit bowed and my heart low. But having realized my true purpose, these things had somehow faded into the background as "just my life."

Just my life? Yes. Everybody and I mean everybody in life has stuff or "life" to deal with. My stuff was a body that didn't function and was in constant pain. There are equal or greater challenges. There are single parents with hungry mouths to feed. There are so many souls in way less fortunate circumstances than me. If I thought about it for too long, I could convince myself I was positively blessed. In truth, I was and I am. The proverbial looking on the bright side perhaps, but perspective and attitude are everything!

There's Nothing Wrong With Me!

This led me to the astounding revelation that there was nothing wrong with me; nothing broken, nothing to be fixed, I was perfect just the way I was.

Don't fall off your couch here; you know how hard it is to get back up!

How could I possibly say such a thing?

Perhaps it was my disease-ridden brain, but I wondered if the same people, seeing me in a wheelchair for example, would give me a hard time for not having found a way to walk again? Wouldn't it be more appropriate to congratulate such a person for finding a way to live their fullest life possible while managing very challenging life circumstances, rather than suggesting I was somehow deficient in areas I hadn't even contemplated!

So instead of listening to all I had done wrong, I congratulated myself for suiting up and showing up to the best of my ability and magic started to happen.

Playing My Way

I reasoned the only time I felt deficient in any way was when I tried to play with others and in a way most people did. So long as I stayed with the things I knew I could do, however slowly and painfully, I could achieve much, kind of the tortoise and the hare idea.

I had already looked at other people and realized my life looked nothing like theirs. I was not in a position to work or play like them, but play I could, my way! I stopped trying to create energy to work because that was putting the cart before the horse. It might be what most people did, but I wasn't most people and couldn't play by those rules even if I wanted to.

Instead of my life being a series of disappointments and frustrations at all I had lost and could no longer do, it started to become a celebration of all the little things I *could* do. When I took the time to look at that, I realized I had somehow become a person who got things done.

When and how did that happen!

So I now have a reason to be here. I have figured out I have a purpose and what that is and now I'm achieving things. I'm still physically challenged, but really good things are starting to happen. What is going on?

Bringing Step One Together

Though we haven't talked a bit about food, nor speculated about what could be wrong or which specialist you should seek help with next, you now have a plan. You have a way to move forward and you know exactly who is going to get you there.

You!

Take time to congratulate yourself on how far you have come in the first few pages of this book. Dare to imagine what may be possible by the end! It may seem like nothing much has happened, but a subtle shift has taken place within you. You are open and receptive to recovery, however that may look for you.

After years of feeling sick and worn out to the very core of your being, you are beginning to see what you have endured and overcome and rather than lament and beat yourself up for all you cannot do and have failed to achieve, you give yourself a hug. For the first time, you see your strength and determination and the courage you have shown in dealing with your devastating condition.

In the spirit of all good health and wellness sessions, I'm going to give you a summary of what we covered and a couple of recommendations as you move forward. I'll talk more about the magic that can happen when you work with a professional health coach in a later chapter, but for now, here's what is important.

1. Know with all your being that whatever your contribution to this world, it is important, as are you. Just because you can't play like others does *not* mean you don't have a purpose.
2. If all you are able to do is contribute to the good thoughts of the world, that is not only purpose enough, but also the kind of action that has the power to change not only you but the entire world!
3. Congratulate yourself for your courage and tenacity in facing and dealing with your particular set of challenging life circumstances. So many would have withered under the weight. Not only have you hung in there, you are doing life *YOUR* way!
4. Read the following chapter on Chronic Disease. I've kept the boring stuff to a minimum, but a brief look at the underpinnings of all chronic disease will be helpful as we move forward through the other steps.

I leave you with this quote.

"You'll never be successful until you turn your pain into greatness, until you allow your pain to push you from where you are to where you need to be. Stop running from your pain and embrace your pain. Your pain is part of your prize, a part of your product. I challenge you to push yourself.

Eric Thomas

CHAPTER 2

Chronic Disease, The Modern Day Pandemic

The Most Common Chronic Diseases and their costs to society and us

Though this will be a thankfully brief chapter, I think it's important to understand how so many of us have found ourselves chronically sick. We live in what I call the perfect storm, with so many challenges to human health; a good case can be made for each challenge being *the* culprit and reason for our dilemma.

But we don't live in a world like that do we? Everything, we are discovering, is connected to everything else and it isn't possible to make one change and it not affect a myriad of other things.

This principle works in your favor when tackling what seems the insurmountable task of repairing your health. Making a change in one area of your life will have an effect on many others and so a series of small steps makes it possible for exponential change to occur with relatively little effort.

Back to the depressing subject of being sick.

The toxic chemical soup we all swim in, that we'll cover in Chapter Four, challenges our immune systems which is the very thing that protects us from what can be a hostile world, requiring more energy to keep us healthy. We look for increased energy in the foods we eat, but the mass-produced, processed items considered foods in the Standard American Diet are often so devoid of nutrition, they need to be fortified with chemicals.

The base materials to make these products are grown in fields of chemicals from plants modified by even more chemicals and sprayed with yet more chemicals to make sure nothing eats them before they are harvested and put on plates for our consumption.

Convenience, not nutrition has become the norm and we have all paid a heavy price for it. Lack of nutrients plays havoc with an already compromised immune system. The very thing that should fuel our lives robs us of the precious energy we seek by eating it, leaving us deficient of nutrients and starving, often in bodies that become ever larger, despite all our best efforts.

The door is now wide open for disease to stroll in and make its home in our body. It affects so many of us, in fact, having at least one disease ensures you will always be in the company of at least half the population of this country.

We classify these conditions by names; the autoimmune diseases of arthritis, lupus, MS, or the metabolic diseases of obesity, metabolic syndrome or diabetes. Perhaps it's heart disease or cancer that touches the lives of just about every person in this country to one degree or another. Or maybe you're one of the millions who suffer from digestive issues, chronic fatigue syndrome or fibromyalgia.

How much has all this cost us?

As a society, we spend approximately 2.5 trillion dollars on healthcare each year, yet:

65% of Americans are overweight.
More than 30% of our children have Type 2 Diabetes.
45% of the population has at least one chronic disease.
Chronic disease is responsible for:
7 out of 10 deaths
81% of hospital admissions
76% of doctors' visits and
91% of all prescriptions[1]

---

1   http://www.cdc.gov/chronicdisease/overview/index.htm

Cardiovascular disease, including heart disease and stroke, is the leading cause of death accounting for almost one in three deaths each year.

Cancer, the second leading cause of death claims more than 500,000 lives every year.[2]

Arthritis, the most common cause of disability, limits activity for 29 million Americans.

Two and a half trillion dollars is a lot of money to pay for such dysfunction, but how much has it cost each person who has had their life stolen by disease?

The cost of losing my life, as I knew it and the ability to function in any meaningful way is incalculable. Fortunately, on the other side of chronic disease, I spend little time on such thoughts. Financially, a rough estimate of my earning ability multiplied by the number of years I was sick, plus the huge amount of out of pocket expenses puts the total figure of maintaining my diseased lifestyle at a very conservative and staggering $600,000.

The fact that these conditions turn out to be mostly the result of diet and lifestyle choices was both a shock and a blessing. I'll leave the speculation of why and how we got to this dark place to those who care to discuss such things. Having participated in that myself for many years, I am all about action these days and to that end, let's move on to some answers!

80% of all Chronic Diseases are Diet and lifestyle Related[3]

So just how do diet and lifestyle choices lead to such devastating diseases and what if anything can you do to reverse yours?

The fact that we create these diseases by the diet and lifestyle choices we make is a huge blessing in disguise. That you possibly have within your hands the answer to diseases that have baffled many for decades is really good news, even if it has taken years of devastating illness to get to this point.

For a long time, it seems disease has somehow become the default human condition. Instead of our birthright of optimum health and performance,

---

2 http://www.cdc.gov/nchs/fastats/deaths.htm

we have somehow, somewhere along the line, settled for dysfunction on a massive scale.

When was the last time you heard someone asking why so many are sick and dying? Though that is the truth, it is not what we talk about. We talk instead about the number of medications we take, comparing notes and costs, wearing our disabilities like a right of passage to an old age that starts decades before its time.

One of the reasons I went back to school was to learn the answer to this question and many others. Since I completed my training at the Institute for Integrative Nutrition®, I use my knowledge to practice as a certified health and wellness coach, helping others rediscover their health and passion for life.

I could fill up chapters and chapters with all the reasons so many are chronically sick, yet it would be only more information to add to your already extensive collection of why we are at this point and exactly how we got here. All of great interest, I'm sure, but it is absolutely useless in moving you forward in your goal of getting from the couch to life!

Suffice it to say, much has been done to our food supply and we have sacrificed quality sustenance for convenience at a terrible price. What we call food is often little more than processed commodities with infinite shelf lives, available in endless quantities.

Why have we done this?

In part because we were told it was the way to a happy life, a life where there is no need to stop and take care of one of the most fundamental requirements for human life. Nourishment in the form of food as made by nature, not man. As we have already seen, making a change to one thing affects many others, so the consequences of negating this most basic of needs naturally spilled over into other areas of our lives.

Heck, if we could dispense with the need to feed ourselves nourishing nature made food, who would need to get adequate rest or nurture their soul? It seems all the body, mind and soul food necessary for a healthy, happy life became about speed and convenience and we began to forget the very essence of what nourishes us. Instead of looking at life as a whole, we started to break everything down into its constituent parts, convinced we, man, could reconstitute them at will with results far superior to anything nature could command.

So when our bodies began to break down, there was no longer a whole to return to, no blueprint for us to consult to put us on the right track. Everything was about the parts and how they could be manipulated, improved, perhaps dispensed with altogether.

Medicine has been fractured into parts as well. Doctors for the mind, doctors for the soul and doctors for just about every system in the body you can imagine and then some. All infinitely and exquisitely trained in their respective fields yet each one seeming to lack one essential, vital piece. A blueprint, a map of how we fit together and how each part affects the whole.

Without such a blueprint, the practice of medicine descends into super specialties, requiring ever more knowledge and information to try and answer the question of what is wrong.

Without a blueprint for our lives, it is equally impossible to figure out what could be wrong with us, much less how to start making the necessary changes, even while our answers hover in front of us and we continue looking for it in the pieces.

And you know I don't believe it will ever be possible to find the answer among the pieces. Not to something as complex as human health because it encompass so much more than just our physical bodies and the food we choose to power them with.

Once you separate things into their parts, the number of possibilities become overwhelming, making any reasonable attempt at answers, much less action, impossible. The answer to what each part needed for my health to be restored seemed something I would take to my grave!

So how about medicines and all the wonderful drugs that have literally saved the lives of millions? Haven't we all tried our fair share of these? We hear every day how they can take care of so many of our symptoms, but if that were true, not one person would need to read this book. We would all be too busy living the lives we know we are supposed to be living!

In the next pages, we'll look at what medicines really do to us and how much we pay to delude ourselves into thinking they are a quick, easy fix.

Medicine is Not Always The Answer

Let me first say that medicine has saved the lives of millions and absolutely has a place in treating disease. It seems so obvious it isn't worth the space these words take up, but I want to make that clear before I cover some very frightening facts about what medications can really do to us.

We've all heard those commercials that tell us about the latest wonder drug and how it will enable us to start living our lives again. It is closely followed by a long, long list of all the things that might happen if you take it.

One thing people don't always appreciate is that all drugs have an effect. We label some effects beneficial and a solution and others, side effects. The message is always that the benefits of the "effects" far outweigh the "side effects."

We are often told and wholeheartedly believe no other changes to our lives are required for a return of our health, so it makes this an enormously attractive solution to our problems.

But what price are we really paying with this option?

An estimated 450,000 medication-related adverse events occur in the US every year.

Medications, even when taken as prescribed, are the third leading cause of death in the US.[3]

For the first time in history, the number of deaths from medications now exceeds those killed in traffic accidents.[4]

As I say, I am a firm believer in the need and efficacy of medications in treating many diseases, but not for those created by diet and lifestyle choices. In fact, I think it is a completely irresponsible practice of medicine to continue

---

3 Lazarou J, Pomeranz BH, Corey PN. Incidence of adverse drug reactions in hospitalized patients: a meta-analysis of prospective studies. JAMA. 1998 Apr 15;279(15):1200-5. http://www.cdc.gov/media/pressrel/2010/r100617.htm

4 http://articles.latimes.com/2011/sep/17/local/la-me-drugs-epidemic-20110918

prescribing a potentially fatal remedy that will only mask symptoms, when a real and lasting cure is within easy reach.

Yes, easy reach. Maybe not a seemingly instant answer, but within the grasp of anyone who wants to understand their beautiful unique selves and how to fuel that self with the delicious foods of life that nourish their body, mind and soul.

Think about it. As attractive as the instant fix sounds, I don't believe any of us are looking for health. No. We're looking for all the things health can bring us, all the things it will allow us to do in life, with the boundless energy that has been relegated to a distant memory, if not our dreams. How can one pill, however cleverly designed and crafted possibly deliver anything close to that?

We're Living Longer but in Poorer Health

I marvel at the resiliency of the human body and the sheer amount of abuse it can take and still keep ticking. It is a true miracle and testament to this incredible biological system.

I say this as a person who has tested my body to its absolute limits and beyond. The details of this abuse are enough to fill another book. Lets just say, I put up both my hands and confess that I took the medications and kept right on abusing my body. I neglected its care in just about every way possible until it finally brought me to my knees and forced me to pay attention.

I told you in the first chapter how small my life became when I lost my health and how it impacted every aspect of my life. Though I was taking eight medications, they were barely enough to help me function and the strongest of the medications could only take the edge off my pain.

The best combination of drugs from the best that medicine had to offer only succeeded in keeping me sick and tired. I was trapped in a broken body with no hope of recovery. That was not a life that made any sense to me.

Beginning my journey to health made me challenge the current thinking about my medical condition. Determined to find a way, I pushed myself to find answers, reasoning that if such an effort killed me before my time as was predicted, I would at least have given it my best shot. I told myself and believed with all my heart, I'd rather live ten years of such a life than thirty in chronic pain, sickness and despair.

Besides, I had come a long way from those dark and desperate hours. Against the odds and creating my blueprint as I went, I had pulled myself up and was starting to consider a life off my couch, daring to dream about life outside my home. Step by step, I had found a reason and purpose for life and I was hungry for more. I couldn't help wondering how much better I could function, how much bigger my life could be if I were in the optimum conditions to thrive?

I was about to find out!

CHAPTER 3

Your Road To Recovery – A New Blueprint for Health

Now you've taken that all-important first step, it's time to roll up your sleeves and start tackling your own unique health challenge. We have the boring stuff out of the way and understand how our diets and lifestyle choices not only play a part in our chronic illness but are also in fact the primary driving force. We have looked at what it does to a human being to have their life, as they know it, taken from them and what it might take to even contemplate a move from the couch.

We've looked at the medications currently used to "manage" these conditions and realized that not only are drugs not the answer, they mask symptoms while the underlying disease marches on unchecked in people completely unaware they are ticking time bombs.

So now what?

You're almost ready to take on your diet but before you do.....

I talked in Chapter One about "Playing Your Way" and suggested that as long as you don't try and compete with others (you wish!), you could never fail.

Having been so used to beating myself up for not being able to play like others, my newfound understanding of the sheer courage and determination it had taken to make it this far, fanned the flames of that little light.

The warmth of its glow started to penetrate my body, lighting up parts that had been asleep so long, I had forgotten they existed.

My mind had suffered terribly. Surgery to remove a benign brain tumor in 2005 did get rid of the migraines, so intense, sunglasses covered with a towel in a dark room still let in so much light, my eyes felt like they were being pierced with red hot needles. But a low-grade pain remained behind them, making driving in bright sun or headlights at night increasingly difficult.

A throbbing pain that I can only describe as intense pressure followed activity that was remotely strenuous, including any attempt at focused thinking for longer than a few minutes. Processing information at any speed was enormously challenging and impacted my life in many ways.

Daily household tasks took on obsessive-compulsive proportions. By the time I had completed a task, I had forgotten half of what I had done and had to constantly recheck everything to make sure it was compete. I began avoiding these tasks that challenged me and took so much of my precious energy.

The anxiety of driving, even in our small town with a handful of stoplights and a speed limit of 25 mph became so exhausting and frightening, I all but hung up the keys. By the time I'd looked all ways at a four way stop and processed whether there were any cars, one would invariably appear and start the whole process again. I began to go miles out of my way to make sure I only had to turn at a stoplight.

Some days, my head felt so fried, I wouldn't even attempt to drive. I would literally tell my husband, "this is a no driving day today," which often turned into more days, then weeks as I fought to restore some kind of balance.

In reality, there was nothing to do accept retire yet again to the couch and wait for the dizziness to stop, for the fog to clear, for the pain in my body to diminish and for some energy to return. Always I looked for an answer to one of the biggest challenges I had ever faced in my life and always, it remained out of reach.

I remembered it was my mind that had pulled me from the depths of despair and launched me on this journey, so it seemed reasonable it could maybe get me to the next stage, whatever that might be.

In a wonderful display of synchronicity, I was about to be provided with an opportunity to test my theory!

I had joined an online community of people who seemed to have the same symptoms as me. All were just as baffled, had lost their functioning lives to one degree or another and were looking for answers. Though none were available, it was such a relief to know there were others just like me in the world.

For the first time in years, I felt connected to something and my tiny, tiny world became a little larger.

The community was and still is run by a wonderful gentleman called Daniel Moricoli, who had poured hours and hours of his time and thousands upon thousands of dollars, building an online community so we could connect, share stories, information, encouragement and find some much needed solace. Exploring the site one day, I came across a little paragraph and my heart skipped a beat. "Volunteers Needed. This site is run by volunteers and any assistance and time you could donate would be much appreciated," or words to that effect.

Could I do this?

"Don't be ridiculous," came the instant reply, "you can barely put one thought in front of the other," yet somehow, my fingers were typing out the words, "I'm not sure how I can possibly help, but I am willing to volunteer and help with the site." I stared at the words in the email for a long time, my heart beating ever harder until it leapt into my mouth as I hit the send button.

Oh my goodness, what have you done now?

Pushing Through

It was such a delight to meet Daniel and connect with a fellow soul who was doing everything he could to help himself and anyone else struggling with this devastating illness. The name Chronic Fatigue hardly begins to describe a dysfunction that includes the immune system and just about every other system in the human body. Again, know I share my story so you may recognize yourself in it and know that at least for one other person in the world with a similar condition, recovery was possible.

Daniel and I had similar stories. Even though neurological dysfunction was on Daniel's top ten list of debilitating symptoms, he found a way to work with it to create this amazing community. I was impressed, grateful and in awe.

It helped that from day one he understood my challenges. He knew from his own experience there was often days, perhaps weeks, occasionally months, when the brain would not play ball. Just getting through a day was often too challenging, so trying to corral it into doing something as intense as helping build an online community was often out of the question.

Little by little, by showing up when I could, nurturing myself when I was sick and congratulating myself for even attempting to stretch and challenge such a dysfunctional mind, I noticed big changes happening and my hard work and perseverance started to pay big dividends.

I felt something long dormant in me come to life. Was it hope? Was it perhaps the belief that somehow, crazy as the thought was, I might actually have created a viable life for myself, despite my devastating condition?

What had I done to move myself from feeling useless to having purpose and a reason to get up in the morning?

Could it really have been as simple as showing up, volunteering and giving my broken, dysfunctional self to others for whatever use I could be to them?

Is this the principle of giving and receiving at work?

So many questions; were there ever any answers to be found?

Start Right Where You Are

We ended the last section with a series of questions, so this one starts with some answers, at least, my answers!

On the surface, it may seem all I did was stubbornly refuse to give into my mind's dysfunction, but what so often looks like a simple act, in this case of defiance, can often conceal important underlying principles at work.

Just as the rest of our body replaces itself on a regular basis, old, unused connections in the mind are broken and new ones formed. Again, this is great news. It means that with focus, we can literally rewire our minds. This is another way we see the mind/body connection in action.

Rewiring the mind provides us with new opportunities that change our perspective. This affects our mood that drives our emotions that determines how we perceive and react to the world that in turn determines our experience. I deliberately wrote that last sentence as an unashamed run-on sentence to demonstrate how impossible it is to separate things into parts. Each flows seamlessly into the other.

That's what I believe I did. I acknowledged that large parts of my head were not working. Instead of trying to fix them, I used my energy to rewire my head to bypass the broken parts.

Had I sat and thought how I might accomplish such a task, my brain may have spontaneously combusted with the effort, but this is one of the enormous benefits of hindsight, so often seen as a negative, unhelpful reflection.

What did hindsight tell me about what I did?

It told me I chose to look for another way to use my mind, to whatever extent that was possible, and in doing so, created a new pathway, one that could actually accomplish this task. Cool huh?

This new ability, after feeling like a failure for so long, completely changed my ideas and beliefs of what may be possible for my life. It moved me from a place of needing answers in order to move forward, to moving forward, knowing the answers would appear.

I could repeat what I said above about how one small change creates a ripple effect in our lives and leads to enormous changes, but instead, I want to talk briefly about treatments before we tackle the subject of bringing life back to a much needed whole so the ripple effort has exponential benefits to our health and well being.

So where are you right now, at this moment?

What is one thing, just one thing you could do that might start creating a new pathway for you?

If focus is a challenge, ask yourself what tiny step you could take to improve your focus. Does it mean reading one paragraph a day, even if it means you spend the rest of the day sleeping with exhaustion?

Will you give yourself the gift of space and time to show up again and again, despite what feels like a gazillion attempts that end in perceived failure? Will you be patient and allow what looks like setbacks to do their thing? They will create an all-important new pathway.

When I was going through the process, I would often think of Edison and each time I felt I had failed, I would remind myself I was one step closer to the answer. In case you're not familiar with the story, Edison was always adamant he had not once failed in his attempts to produce the first electric light bulb; he just uncovered more than a thousand ways it didn't work! That's the kind of perspective and perseverance I'm talking about.

Can you imagine how it would feel to have accomplished such a thing?

Let's look at how one small, tiny baby step can set this powerful change in motion.

Bringing Your Life Back To A Whole

One of the many challenges of chronic illness is it separates you into so many pieces. Flying to the moon feels far more doable than understanding each piece, much less attempting to figure out what each piece might need for health to return.

Referred to different specialists for different body systems, it is easy to slip down a rabbit hole without even knowing it, finding yourself in the strange and enormously expensive land of medical specialties.

Here is a perfect example of how that works, but first let me say, with one or two notable exceptions, every doctor I have seen has only had my best interests at heart and has done their absolute best to help me. What I'm about to say isn't a reflection of inadequate medical care; far from it; but the consequence of living in a world that has reduced everything to those maddening parts we talked about earlier.

Excuse the personal nature of what I'm about to share, but when my digestive system went awry, I was referred to gastroenterologists. After many invasive and costly tests, this was the conclusion. "Your digestive system is dysfunctional."

No kidding; that's why I came to see you!

What followed was a series of drug interventions designed to take over my dysfunctional digestive system. My acid pumps were shut off, I was given digestive enzymes, barbiturates to slow my whole system down, the kind of gel you usually see in diapers was prescribed for fiber; the list went on and on. There was no way my body could figure out which way was up if it tried.

During all these tests and consultations, there was no discussion of food, intolerances or suggestions of dietary changes. How bizarre that the fuel which transits our digestive tracts isn't the first place to look when things go wrong. Like not checking the fuel gauge when your car runs out of power!

This is a perfect example of how fracturing things into parts make it impossible to see the forest for the trees. It isn't possible to separate anything into its different parts and understand how the whole works by studying each one. In fact, it seems the more each one is studied, the more elusive answers become.

Remember Mary Shelley's *Frankenstein*? However carefully the most perfectly selected part was added to another, nothing approaching a human being could be created. Not all the care, knowledge or concern in the world could change the fact that even though all the components were present, something very fundamental was missing.

We see this with food too. We look at broccoli for example and say; well, it contains these substances; minerals, vitamins, fiber; so if we put those together in a lab and compress it into a pill, people can take that and not be concerned with the food they eat. Their nutritional requirements have been taken care of. And clever them, not wasting time or money buying and preparing expensive food. This is the 21st Century; who has time for that?

On closer inspection, we see that the magical missing ingredient in "broccoli pills" for example, is in fact, broccoli. Somehow, nature has found a way of combining certain nutritional components in little packages called vegetables and however hard we try, we just cannot best her!

Trying to separate food in this way makes it totally impossible to work out whether you are eating the right food in the right quantities, whether you've covered all your bases, whether all your wonderful systems have been nourished and have all they need. With so many variables, it is impossible to make the simplest of decisions about what to eat, much less the bigger questions in life!

This imbalance spills over into every area of our lives.

Encouraged to consider every last detail of our lives, the sheer number of decisions that have to be made often paralyses us. No wonder we never feel we achieve our goals!

The only way to restore sanity is to bring your life back to a whole. Lets take a deep breath and gain some much need clarity. Instead of constantly trying to work out what nutrition all your parts need, how about something radical yet simple.

Put food and nourishment at the very core of your life.

Whether the kind we eat or the kind we feed our minds in the form of thoughts, nutrition in all its forms is central to our health and wellbeing. If you were to make that and only that the focus of your life, how vibrantly nourished might all areas of your life feel?

Instead of looking at all your parts and what they need, putting nutrition at the core of your life and all you do will transform everything.

Simple. Easy.

You can use this technique to bring yourself back to a whole anytime you feel yourself fractured. Define what's central to all the parts, make it the core of everything and watch as your life comes into balance. Now it's easy to see what is needed and you will never again get lost in the detail.

Once I had pulled my fractured self back to a whole the next steps became so obvious, I almost tripped over them. I knew I needed wholesome food, water, rest and a connection to my community. I needed to play my part, however small, in making my community a better place, even if that was only in the thoughts I contributed.

So nourishment became my core and I looked at what was in most need of nourishing. Clearly it was my body, so that was that was my starting point. So long as I focused solely on nutrition, the whole of me would benefit. If I focused instead on one section of the whole, all of me would suffer. Nutrition could be one or a combination of "foods," for my body, mind, soul or larger life in my community.

Sounds complicated, but what it meant was switching to whole organic foods, making them the basis of my diet and removing the toxins from my environment. I put myself on a media diet to help keep me sane, kept watch over my thoughts and began volunteering. On the couch or on your feet, all of this is within your reach.

Connecting my mind and body in this way made my path much clearer. Any change I made had an impact on all areas of my life and I stopped seeing myself as a fractured, separated entity. Changes in my thoughts and food gave me the energy and strength I needed to look at my situation differently.

Those small changes were all that was necessary to begin seeing how all the elements of my life had contributed to my sickness. Turning my listening inward, I heard the sweet symphony of my body for the first time, effortlessly working and being alive.

Naomi Remen says, "Our listening creates a sanctuary for the homeless parts within another person." I can see how listening to my body is what brought all my homeless pieces together at last.

My life experiences have shown me there is rarely just one answer for anything. Life is anything but black and white. Instead of looking for the answer among all those maddening parts, I realized I was a whole, complete person with one over-riding need. Nourishment.

I may have needed many different forms of nourishment, for body, mind and spirit, but identifying nutrition as the issue, then looking at all the ways I need to nourish my life is what helped me become whole again.

CHAPTER 4

Taking Action

Give yourself the Biggest Gift of Your Life – A Licensed Health and Wellness Coach

Give yourself the biggest gift possible and find a health and wellness coach certified in Integrative Nutrition® to work with. Trained in hundreds of dietary theories, they are familiar with the part that our diets and lifestyles play in driving the chronic diseases which are robbing us of our lives. More importantly, they can teach you the necessary life skills to do in months what it took me years to do. Had I known such people existed during my long journey back to health, I would have done all I could to track one down and shorten my journey!

To write a fully comprehensive book on the techniques a health and wellness coach trained in Integrative Nutrition® might employ in moving you from where you are to where you want to be, would turn this book into an epic. Even if all the techniques *could* be covered, it still would not help you move forward. As we already know, lack of information is not and never has been our problem.

They are what I call the How-To Manuals for life, and once you have learned the techniques that work specifically for your life, you can use them at will to create and overcome whatever life may throw at you.

Let me be clear about something. When I talk about "overcoming" health conditions, I am not necessarily talking about a complete return to what we usually define as health, though that is the goal and within reach for many. Sometimes, just as we will never all be a size six, recovery may mean a different outlook on our circumstances; one that allows us to lift our heads above the cloud of depression caused by a life relegated to the couch. It may not mean we escape its physical confines, but certainly, soaring above its mental confines is achievable for most.

Health is defined in many ways, only one of which is physical; so don't write yourself off because that may not be achievable for you. That would be to deny the wholeness of who you are. Perhaps the idea that all depends on an ability to function physically is part of what holds many back from total health.

This setback and many others are exactly the kind of thing a health and wellness coach is trained to help you overcome with easy to implement skills. Moving forward can be quick, easy and painless.

Yes, I am a health and wellness coach, certified in Integrative Nutrition® so of course I'm going to promote the skills myself and others like me can provide. But honestly, it is what the certification represents that is important.

I had managed to get myself a long way on my own but it was a long, slow, often agonizing process. I groped and felt my way along, taking many wrong turns and dead ends. So many times I gave up in despair, refusing to "play" at life at all until my sense of humor returned from wherever it had been hiding and I was ready to try again. Depending on the challenge and setbacks I encountered, that could be weeks, or months.

I enrolled at the Institute for Integrative Nutrition® because I wanted to know how and why what I had done worked and how I might take my health to the next level. Having made enormous leaps by changing my approach to my illness, my life, the choices I had made up to that point and the food I chose to fuel my body with, I wanted to tune out the ever louder noise of what we should and shouldn't be eating.

Just the relief in taking that step released a ton of energy that had been consumed by trying to follow and understand the latest media generated thinking on nutrition. I will never forget the day I enrolled, almost a year ago to the day of writing this book. The frustration of trying to sift through and decipher the mass of information before I could determine if it was of use to me finally became too much.

Pushed by some invisible force, I leapt out of the bath, picked up the phone and enrolled on the spot. The date? Friday, December 21, 2013 and the relief was enormous!

I have not looked back. Putting myself on the same program I take all my clients through, I not only transformed my life, I learned the vital skills needed to navigate the many changes our lives inevitably meet.

I had no idea twelve months of study and applying what I learned would bring me to this point. Still having to allow recovery time to do the things I wanted when I enrolled, I was a little concerned that I wouldn't be able to keep up. That seems such a long time ago, I can scarcely believe I am talking about myself. It has been a whole year since I was stopped in my tracks and had to retire to the couch. A whole year!

Of course, it is no coincidence my ability to stay off the couch happened as I started to apply the principles of what I was learning. Having figured out how to get off the couch, my studies began to teach me how to stay off.

I am covering a lot of techniques in this book so with a decent and consistent effort, you can make enormous strides in improving your health as you go from couch to life. As I said at the beginning of this chapter, giving yourself the biggest gift of your life by finding a health and wellness coach will take months off your journey.

If you're the kind of person who needs to work these things out for yourself, there is a good chance you are also a health and wellness coach, so give yourself an even bigger gift. Enroll in the Institute for Integrative Nutrition®, earn your qualifications, and then teach others how to turn their lives around. With chronic disease affecting more than half of us, your skills are badly needed!

Whatever Your Chronic Illness, The Treatment Is The Same

In a minute, we'll be talking about how to increase your energy levels so you can start to tackle your illness. Before we jump into that, I want to share with you that whatever name has been given to your chronic illness, the treatment is the same. There is a set of steps everyone needs to take on their journey to health but the details and order of those steps will be different for each of us. With the exception of the first step, cleaning up your diet and lifestyle.

It isn't necessarily the chronic illness that has taken your function away that will determine the course of your journey to health, but where you most need to start. So the treatment is the same; you determine the order and starting point. Again, this is something a health and wellness coach can help you figure out very quickly.

It has taken me a series of steps to get off the couch and stay off consistently. In fact, my health has now improved to such an extent, it is impossible to distinguish me from those we consider a picture of vibrant health. Because I am a picture of vibrant health!

For me, the steps looked like this, though because the health improvements I gained by changing the food I was eating were so enormous, I would move it up to number one. It is after all the fuel that powers us, and the medicine that heals us.

1. Understanding the meaning of my chronic illness ridden life on the couch.
2. Discovering I not only had purpose, but an important purpose even in that condition.
3. Installing a much-needed mental software upgrade so I could understand the language of, "recovery is possible."
4. Creating a Blueprint for Health.
5. Pushing through my limitations to create new pathways to bypass the dysfunctional parts of my brain.
6. Cleaning up my diet. Later in this chapter.
7. Creating much needed energy; also later in this chapter.
8. Enrolled in the Institute for Integrative Nutrition® to take my health to the next level.

Are these the steps and the order you need to tackle them?

As I said, cleaning up my diet was not the first step I took on my journey, but it did have the biggest impact. Though the journey is yours to make, you do need a few tools to begin.

Clean up your diet first and for the first time in years, you'll start to feel the brain fog lifting. Then you'll be able to install the much-needed mental software that allows you to see recovery is possible. If you stop short of installing it, your outdated software will constantly interfere with your progress, creating doubt and paralyzing fear, making progress difficult and challenging.

So the treatment is the same for everyone with chronic illnesses, the details and starting points are different for all of us. A health and wellness coach can dramatically shorten the time it takes you to work out the best place for you to start and to designing your unique "Blueprint for Health."

Now you have your own blueprint in hand, it's time to create some much-needed energy so you can begin to tackle your specific chronic illness.

Taking Action – Create More Energy

Who couldn't use more energy?

From the fittest to those with the most exhausting chronic health conditions, more energy is good, especially when it has the added bonus of allowing you to make diet and lifestyle changes that further enhance your health. This is the ripple effect that allows a series of small steps to take us exponentially further.

Though food is a large part of creating more energy, it can equally have the opposite effect. Instead it can suck the remaining vestiges of energy from us while leaving us malnourished and devoid of the materials we need to repair our broken bodies, minds and spirits.

Who could get off the couch under those circumstances?

I still remember the days when the thought of having to walk to the mailbox each day would fill my whole day with anxiety. The thought of the exhaustion that would ensue was enough to make me ill. As soon as my eyes opened in the morning, I would start fretting about how I was going to find the energy to do it. I knew exactly how many steps it was from door to box; sixty; one hundred and twenty steps round trip.

Then there were the 'girls," our chickens that needed feeding and locking up at night to keep them safe from the coyotes. The animal rounds would start around 4pm. Dogs, a cat, chickens, resident ducks and wild birds, all needed feeding and it was totally exhausting! The number of paces from back door to chicken coop was thirty, round trip sixty steps.

Then there were the bathroom visits. This is when I really learned to rehabilitate my bladder. I minimized the amount of fluid I drank just so I didn't have to spend energy walking to the bathroom. Even though it was only fifteen steps from couch to bowl, it was a trip I wanted to make the least number of times possible.

This section is about creating energy and though that does involve food, it does not contain details of specific diets. Rather, it includes steps and techniques you can use to complete your journey of recovery. The details of specific diets can be found on my website and you'll find some great recipes at the end of this book to get you started.

Look at it as a prescription for working out where you are and how to get to where you want to be. The details of the journey, the roads you'll take? That's all up to you. But any journey needs fuel, so lets looks at some ways you can increase your energy with a few simple steps. For the details, look at the resources I provide in the back.

Is it possible to create more energy? Of course is the simple answer!

Food is an obvious way, but maybe in more ways than you may have considered. Making a few changes in this area can bring immediate relief and you may find yourself surprised by what can happen in a short space of time. Requiring little more than making some changes in preparing and eating the food that fuels your life, these changes will help you save money in many ways.

As I cleaned up my diet, my symptoms began to fade one by one and I found I no longer needed some of my medications. Over an eight-month period, I stopped my medications one by one, saving more than $4,000 a month.

But back to energy.

Lack of energy can make us reach for the very things that will deplete our energy even further. Our drive for energy is so strong, willpower is no match for a body in need of fuel. The things we reach for can end up costing us more energy than they deliver, so the very first way to generate some much-needed energy is to eat whole food, as grown by nature, not man. Why eat whole food? There are so many reasons!

Ten Extra Energy Points Plan

Eat Whole Food

As I mentioned earlier, nature has conveniently packaged food, in things like vegetables and fruit and these packages contain, in addition to important vitamins, minerals and fiber; live enzymes that help us break down the food. With enzymes already present, your body doesn't need to produce as many, so you've just released some energy. Lets say:

- 1 Point -

NOTE: Cooking food over a certain temperature destroys these precious enzymes; so adding raw foods can make a big difference. Cooking your veggies is still okay, in fact, a good idea. Cooking destroys some elements while making others available, so don't think you have to reduce yourself to munching on lettuce leaves and raw carrots the rest of your life.

If you are not currently eating whole foods, then adding them, raw and cooked, will give your health a huge boost, so it's still one point!

Whole food is unprocessed

What I love about nature made food is, apart from a quick rinse under the tap to wash off the dirt, perhaps a quick scrub of the skin, they are ready to eat. Though there are tons of ways to enhance them further, eating them just as they are goes a long way to bringing your life back to a whole again. Corny to say that eating whole foods helps you bring things back to a whole? I don't think so. Chapter six talks about this in more detail.

Without having to deal with the devastating effects processed foods can have on our health, robbing us of precious energy rather than replenishing our stores, I'm going to give this two points; one for providing first class fuel for the body and one for not having the food you're eating suck the life out of you!

- 1 Point -

Eat Super foods
Some foods come complete with everything our body needs and eating such food gives us a full spectrum of nutrients. These are called super foods. You will find a list of them in the resources section of this book, along with some simple recipes so you can start using them straight away.

Some superfoods come from different parts of the world. Maca for example, comes from South America, the mighty Gogi berry from Asia and raw cacao from South America, parts of Africa and the Philippines.

Spirulina, a blue green algae, is a complete protein and can be grown almost anywhere, its location dictating its specific nutritional profile. By weight, it is approximately sixty to seventy percent protein and is often compared to meat and the mighty kale in terms of its protein content.

It is packed with B vitamins, iron, antioxidants and important fatty acids. Though few would advise it, it is said a person can live on spirulina and water alone. It does have a very satisfying, satiating effect because it is a complete protein and full of other great nutrients, which is great if you want to contain your appetite.

Close to home and right in front of many of us, are things like blueberries, cranberries, hemp seeds, broccoli, and the mighty kale.

Eating super foods can give you a real boost in energy. When I drink my kale smoothie with blueberries and spirulina, I literally feel my body coming alive. Knowing that the effects of adding simple super foods to your diet will be so impressive, you'll add at least two of them, I'm going to give this:

- 2 Points -

See how one simple change can have a big impact. What could you do with four extra energy points, just by changing the way you eat? When was the last time you had the luxury of such a problem?

The Non-Toxic Life

I'm going to try and give a brief summation of what I call, "*the Non Toxic Life.*" You can read about the details on my website and find all the resources you need to make these changes, step by easy step, but I want to give you an overview of why switching to a non-toxic life is so important.

We are swimming in a sea of chemicals.

From our food, grown in soil soaked in chemical fertilizer, dowsed in chemical pesticides or worse still, impregnated with chemicals so plants can manufacture them directly, our bodies have to cope with a massive amount of toxic substances.

We use chemicals to stop clothes from catching on fire and douse our furniture with more chemicals so they don't get dirty. We put toxic chemicals on our body in the form of body care products, store our food in dangerous plastics, worse still, zap them in the microwave and call it dinner.

We toss bleach around as if a sea of the stuff will take care of anything that might "harm us" while paying no attention to the fact using it is harming just about everything on the planet, including us!

Toxic cleaners and manufactured fragrances make our homes smell wonderful, while destroying our lungs, our immune systems and our animals who live much closer to the ground than us. Okay, not us specifically, unless you have one of those fancy, elevated couches, but you get the point!

We are surrounded by so many chemicals it seems impossible to escape their toxic cloud and with many companies making expensive natural alternatives, going with the flow seems way easier.

But before you do, consider this. Your body has to work hard to rid itself of all this stuff. Discussions about whether they cause cancer or have other long-term health implications aren't the point here; the energy your body needs to get rid of them is. The more stuff you ask your body to process, the more energy you will expend.

So forget the discussions about whether they are safe or not, understand they are sucking precious energy from you and stop using them!

Here's how your points look for this:

Buying Organic Food

Fertilizers and pesticides cover our fruits and vegetables, so buying organic where possible will save your body a ton of energy in getting rid of them. The Environmental Working Group (EWG), provides a list called, The Clean 15 and Dirty Dozen, a list of the most and least contaminated produce and you'll find their website in the resource section of this book.

Though this list can save you money, you may want to read "A New Way To Look at Food,'" in Chapter five first and decide whether you want any non-organic produce in your body.

- 1 Point -

Personal Care products are some of the worst offenders for containing things you shouldn't be putting anywhere near your body. Often disguised with names like natural and organic, they are anything but.

The Environmental Working Group are also committed to exposing the toxic chemicals used in the industry. The have a database called, *"The Cosmetics Database,"* where you can enter the products you currently use and it will give you a score from 0 to 10, designating how toxic they may be. A zero is in the green and safe, while a 10 is so toxic, you might want to send it to Hazmat for disposal.

Just kidding, but seriously, this is scary stuff.

Aside from the potential to cause things to go very wrong in the body as many of these chemicals mimic our own hormones, just think about the energy you are wasting, trying to deal with that delicious "organic Shea butter," washed in petroleum and doused in chemical fragrances!

I think I could make a good case for a point for each toxic product you remove from your life, but I may get up into double figures and need my calculator, so lets just leave it at:

- 1 Point -

Get Rid of the Plastic!

Plastics have taken over our lives. I remember my dad telling me way back in the early 1970's when they were just starting to manufacture everything under the sun with this new technology that plastics they would change the world. I don't think he had any idea how right and prophetic he was at the time.

Again, this isn't a discussion about the efficacy of plastics fun though that may be, but about energy. When we use those plastic containers to store our food, chemicals leech out of the plastic into the food and yet again, our body needs to remove them, requiring the very thing we are trying to generate; energy.

This is especially so with acidic foods, like a spaghetti sauce which contain tomatoes, and if you missed the memo that zapping plastic containers in the microwave increases the chemical load exponentially, just stopping this may give you a new lease on life. Switch to glass storage containers and add another:

- 1 Point -

Get Rid of Toxic Cleaners

I mentioned bleach earlier, but it is just one of many toxic chemicals we think nothing of using to keep our homes, clothes and kids clean. I'm not against bleach specifically, but any cleaner full of toxic chemicals that pollute the air in our homes, filling our lungs with chemicals.

Breathing is one of those other necessities for human life, yet we pay no attention to the air we ask our lungs to inhale. Did you know the lungs are one way the body has of getting rid of toxins? How well do you think that will work if the air we are breathing is just as toxic and the stuff our body is trying to throw out?

Thankfully there are many cleaning products now available that don't use such toxic chemicals, but many things you may have around your home can be used to clean. Did you know that the baking soda you use for cooking would also clean your sink? Add some lemon juice and now you have a lime descaler.

You'll find tons of resources on my website, so feel free to use whatever you need. Print it off, use it, refine it, and just stop using all those toxic chemicals!

Getting rid of your toxic chemical cleaners:

- 1 Point -

Exercise

Yes, you did read that right; exercise! How in the world will exercise add energy to your life? Two ways. Let me show you.

The Half Step

Don't be fooled by the simplicity of this action, you will be able to do twice as much with the half step, so what is it and how does it work?

I wish someone had told me about what I call "the half step," way back when I struggled to put one foot in front of the other. Had I known then there was a way to get around that took way less energy; I would likely have become stronger much quicker after I had figured out my diet.

On a hike this summer from South Lake to Long Lake in the glorious Sierra Nevada Mountains, we were getting dressed for our hike when an elderly gentleman hit the trail ahead of us. "Great," I thought, we'll be slowed down, have to stop and chat, when all I wanted to do was start climbing the mountain!

As I watched him, he took small, small steps; about half of one of my strides and that seemed to confirm my thought that he would be slower than the proverbial tortoise. But as I watched, he began to motor up the mountain, never pausing for a second, putting one tiny step in front of the other until he was more than a half mile ahead of us and well out of sight. Really? Bested by an octogenarian? Yep!

I tried his technique and was astounded at how well it worked. The half step as I called it, takes half the energy required for a full stride, conserving energy and allowing you to get into a walking rhythm that reduces energy expenditure even further. I can't explain the feeling of "motoring through," no matter the size of the mountain; little half steps will get you to the top before you know it!

Conserving half your energy with the half step:

- 1 Point -

Bear with me on this next point. It may seem counterintuitive that exercise will give you more energy, just thinking about the energy required to exercise is exhausting right?

The more you vigorously nod in agreement with this statement, the more this may apply to you. When our muscles are exercised and stretched on a regular basic, they start to work much more efficiently and efficiency is key in saving energy.

When we exercise regularly, we help keep our muscles and bones in good shape, so using them actually requires *less* energy to complete the same task as someone who never exercises. We delve into exercise in more detail in chapter six, so for now, just let this point sink in. Exercise period.

- 1 Point -

There you have it.

Eight simple steps, ten additional energy points.

What will you use yours for?

Will you spend more time with family?

Will you use it to rise from your couch and at least change your view?

Will you use it to give yourself a hug and some much needed self-care?

Perhaps a trip out of the house to feel the breeze on your face and smell the scent of a world you thought you'd never play in again?

CHAPTER 5

Your Journey Begins

Man Made Food

Ever since Man took over the feeding of humans and animals on a mass scale, both have become crippled with disease and disability on an enormous scale. This has required ever more medications to try and manage the dysfunction caused by ingesting a diet we were never designed to eat, certainly not for optimal health.

Processed foods made of commodities grown on a mass scale provide the base ingredients for combinations of substances, fortified with man made "nutrients," colored with dyes and flavored to taste like the real thing that most people call food.

To be fair, we have now stuck the word "junk" in front of much of this stuff, and knowing what "junk food" is, is very helpful. But so much still hides disguised in "natural", "good for," "insert health claim," or, "no GMO" remainder of processed products, no wonder most people are confused.

Though no studies have been done to my knowledge, junk does not provide the body, mind or soul with what it needs to be healthy, happy and productive and food is just one example of the junk that has found itself into our every day lives.

The food pyramid we have all followed advises us to consume a diet heavy in grains that, though whole to start with, are anything but by the time they make it into our cereal boxes, loaves of bread and those scary things called "convenience foods."

These foods are the drivers of obesity and diabetes the world is witnessing on a pandemic scale. In fact, there is much evidence that certain foods, processed foods among them, may be behind many of the crippling chronic diseases we see today.

Can It Really Be Our Diet?

Is it truly our diets that are making so many of us sick?

Disease is largely caused by a combination of two things; lack of nutrients and a build up of toxins. This is of course a very over simplified explanation of the myriad causes of disease.

Though genes determine a great many things, it is our physical, mental and emotional environments that switch these genes on or off, determining, in part, whether we are sick or well.[5] Another very over simplified version of a pretty complex process, but our ability to adapt to our environment and pass the information on to our offspring is part of what makes all life, including us, successful.[6] Bruce Lipton does a wonderful job, explaining this in his book, "Biology of Belief."

Lack of nutrients weakens the immune system so disease and infection can proceed unchecked. Toxicity from all the substances we introduce into our bodies builds up, causing inflammation and congestion, the precursors of most chronic diseases.

All is not lost though, not by a long way. Not if by changing your diet and lifestyle, you can get yourself from couch to life, goodness me, no. As we'll see in "Food As Fuel," and "Food as Medicine," there is a simple treatment in the form of delicious, nutritious whole foods.

Health is the default for the human body. We have an innate capacity for high performance but somewhere along the line, we seem to have forgotten that. With all our talk of ailments and medications, anyone listening in on our planet would be convinced dysfunction and disease is our actual birthright.

---

5 Lipton, B. H. 2001 Insight into Cellular Consciousness. Bridges (ISSEEEM Org.) 12(1):5-9

6 https://www.brucelipton.com/resource/article/fractal-evolution

With the amount of time we all spend talking about food, you'd think we'd know what to eat by now. The problem is, we talk about what sounds good, tastes good, what makes us feel good. We don't talk about the energy we need from it or the foods that would help us get through the cold season for example.

We say certain foods are bad for us, though strangely, we often use that label for whole foods, things like bananas for example. We share recipes with friends for triple layer cheesecake, and we clear time in our schedules to make it, but we don't tell people "if you eat this regularly, it will be really bad for you and could lead to chronic disease and disability." Too bad we don't because that could very well be true.

Though we understand such foods are not good choices for health, function and longevity, we just don't talk about it. We know we should eat our veggies, who wasn't told this growing up, but we don't talk about what could happen if we don't eat them.

So why don't we talk about the wonderful benefits of eating food to power our lives?

A New way To Look At Food

Put a seed in some dirt, add a little water and sunshine and the intelligence within it arranges molecules into a mixture of compounds that are high quality nutrient sources for humans.

Whether we are talking of fruits, vegetables, nuts, animal or vegetable protein, all nature made food provides us with way more than the sum of its nutritional components. When we eat food, we exchange information at a cellular level, the molecules in the food connecting and exchanging information with the receptors within our own cells. Our bodies are fed by this and know exactly what to do with the information.

This information is contained in the substances our bodies use to build, repair and rejuvenate us. This is literally how we become what we eat. When we think of food in this way, certain things become clear. It is no longer a surprise that more than fifty percent of the bodies in the US are confused and sick. The information they are receiving from the food they eat makes no sense whatsoever and even worse, there are no translators to help. Deficient in nutrients to start with, this foreign information is useless.

Knowing the very food we eat transmits information about itself to us makes me think a great deal about the kind I want to receive. I certainly don't want the information transmitted by a pesticide, genetically modified organism or lab made substance.

Neither do I want the kind transmitted by meat raised on a concentrated animal feed lot, where cows stand on piles of dirt and manure in the baking hot sun. At least, they do in the Central Valley in California. If you ever want a reality check on how our food is grown and raised, a drive from Bakersfield to Fresno will set you straight, mile after depressing mile.

The frantic energy of penned chickens, living their lives stuffed in a barn with thousands of its fellows, doused in and fed with antibiotics to grow ever bigger and faster; forever looking at the barn door but never the light of day, isn't what I'm looking for either.

How about a pig, tethered to a trough its whole life, unable to move much except its jaws to constantly eat the never-ending food in front of its face until its short life is ended. What kind of information would I be absorbing? Not exactly the stuff that sweet dreams are made of is it?

This is the kind of "food" that feeds our expanding appetites and waistlines and makes dollar meals and endless buffets possible. Contrast this to nature made food.

Seeds bring to mind all the concentrated nutrition and elements needed for new life; enhanced even more by sprouting. Take a minute to imagine how it feels to have the very fundamental building blocks of life coursing through your veins. Is it such a stretch to believe they have the power to rejuvenate and spark new life within you?

When I think about greens, I think of them soaking up the sun, converting its energy into carbohydrates by combining hydrogen with carbon and water; the energy held captive until we consume it and it is released as energy to power *our* lives. From hydrogen surrounding the sun to instant energy coursing through our bodies.

The root vegetables are great storehouses of nutrition, bursting with all that is necessary to sustain life; packaged in such a way that their goodness is released to us over time. Restoring, replenishing, renewing, they provide reserves of energy as deep as their roots.

The Basic Human Diet

Michael Pollan nailed it years ago in his book, "In Defense of Food," and in his later book, "Food Rules," in answer to the question of what we should eat.

"Eat food. Mostly plants. Not too much."

Having studied hundreds of dietary theories across cultures both east, west and in between, I can tell you the optimum diet for the human being is whole foods, largely vegetable based. Across the board, no matter our ancestry, it is the plants that are the common thread. A diet that contains forty percent or more seems to consistently confer good health and vitality.[7] Just as Michael told us. Just as mum and grandma told us!

Contrast this with the fact green vegetables are the most missing food group in the western diet. That's too bad. As I mentioned, processed convenience foods devoid of nutrition make us fat, sore and unwilling, often unable to move from the couch. The nutrients our bodies don't get to repair them and to ward off sickness add fuel to an already smoldering fire. You could almost name your chronic disease under these circumstances.

When I was sick, more than sixty percent of my diet was grain based, and included cereals, breads, pasta; pretty much the standard American diet. The rest was a combination of meat, vegetables, dairy, fruit, and the ubiquitous sugar that always accompanied the refined grains. I had no idea then my diet was making me sick and keeping me on the couch.

---

7   Campbell, TC, Chen J. Diet and chronic degenerative diseases: Perspectives from China. Am J Clin Nutr. 1994;59:1153S–1161S.
Mishra S, Barnard ND, Gonzales J, Xu J, Agarwal U, Levin S. Nutrient intake in the GEICO multicenter trial: the effects of a multicomponent worksite intervention. Eur J Clin Nutr. 2013;67:1066-1071.

Though vegetables and fruit were a daily part of my diet, they accounted for perhaps twenty percent at best, nowhere near enough to power my life at the level I had been living. Nowhere close enough to negate the effects of the lifestyle choices I had made in my half century on this earth!

As I got older, all these stresses collided with years of this diet full of foods that made me sick. The miracle is I found myself on the couch and not six foot under!

It wasn't just the foods I removed that allowed my health to return. Perhaps even more important was what I added in their place. Sixty percent vegetables replaced the sixty percent of grains in my diet.

Many people wonder just how vegetables can turn our physique into a lean, muscled human body. When we think of muscle and obtaining it, we tend to think of slabs of meat rather than the humble vegetable. The truth is, kale is packed with easy to assimilate protein, contains all nine essential amino acids, has more calcium per calorie than milk, and contains one hundred and thirty three percent of our daily vitamin A requirements in a single serving.

There are of course other things your body needs. A good source of protein, either from meat or a vegetarian source; good fats in the form of coconut and olive oils; the details are at the end of this book. The point here is to show you that the basic human diet for optimal health across the globe is vegetable based whole foods.

As Dr. Fuhrman says so eloquently, *"When you eat right, your metabolic rate slows down, you take in more nutrients and less calories. You can maintain your muscle strength, size and physical prowess into later years without having to stuff your mouth with food every 10 seconds.*

Now we know what the optimal diet is for all of us, let's see how we can go further and use food to fuel and power our lives and as medicine to heal what ails us. The Basic Human Diet works across the board for every single human being in every country on every continent. Provided you don't go out and make a bunch of really bad lifestyle choices in celebration, it should keep you free from chronic disease and living a happy, mobile, productive life way into what are sure to be your golden years.

CHAPTER 6

Your Optimal Diet for Recovery

One of the very many things I love about food is that its actions are instant and lasting. What we eat makes us sick or well, happy or sad, not because we like or dislike it, even though that may be true, but because the very things it is made of are either what our bodies need or what makes them more toxic and congested. I don't know about you, but when I get what I need, I'm happy. When I get what I don't want, I'm unhappy. No complex psychological explanations here!

Did you know for example that spirulina, the single cell blue/green algae we talked about in the section on super foods; is a complete food instantly available for use by your cells? Why would you care about that? You're stuck on the couch and read a whole chapter on creating much-needed energy is why.

Packed with an array of B vitamins, heart healthy omega fats, and a slew of other vital vitamins and minerals hard to find on land, this powerhouse provides serious fuel for your day and vital nutrients to replenish your body.

How about the mighty kale? This anti-inflammatory beauty is packed with protein, vitamins, minerals and antioxidants. What might happen if you started your day with the super foods, spirulina and kale? How does that stack up against your processed cereals, even if they are gluten free, fair trade and organic?

We become what we eat and a body given food deficient in what it needs will not function well. If we look at food as the fuel that powers our lives instead, we start to make very different choices. Imagine how you would feel if all, and I mean all of your body's nutritional needs were not just met but exceeded, your body flooded with vibrant, life giving nutrients.

Mother Nature provides us with so much to nourish, replenish, repair and restore our wonderful bodies. Not in vitamins, minerals, carbohydrates, proteins, fats and grains, but as vegetables and fruits, nuts and seeds. They come packaged with all that is needed to make sure they can be digested and absorbed. You might need between 100 and 300mg of vitamin C from a lab made supplement, but when it is packaged in a carrot with hundreds of other powerful antioxidants, 5.3mgs is sufficient. See, Mother Nature, just like her human counterpart, really does know best!

Food as Fuel

Food is the fuel that powers our lives.

Amazing isn't it that so many of us talk about exhaustion while not even considering whether the fuel we are eating is fueling us at all. Many of us crash in the afternoon as our energy levels plummet and in an attempt to give ourselves a boost, we reach for sugary foods full of refined carbs which make the situation a hundred times worse.

We all know it's going to happen yet we do it anyway. It's one of the reasons it's so important to develop a new way of looking at food. Perhaps if we don't have the energy we need, we should change the fuel we are putting in our body.

When we see food as the fuel it is, we can start to make better choices. Instead of what is quick, convenient and tastes good, we can start selecting food based on what we need to get done that day.

A heavy day would need top quality fuel like spirulina, kale, good protein. Later in the day when its time to slow things down, roasted root vegetables would ground us nicely and refuel our stores, just as they do for the plants they were once attached to.

Super foods are so called because they are nutrient dense, antioxidant rich foods that deliver both instant and sustained nutrition with minimal calories. These foods pack a punch and with little preparation, are both nutritious and delicious.

Though it's hard to select just ten, you'll find my list of top ten super foods at the end of this book. I've selected what I call "every day super foods," food that you would not normally think of super in any way because they have such names as broccoli and spinach. True, many of them are the very same ones you likely detested as a child, but you haven't lived until you've tasted broccoli tossed in coconut oil, roasted in a hot oven and sprinkled with sesame seeds. You just haven't!

I was going to painstakingly write out the list of top ten super foods, top ten instant energy foods, slow release, endurance, healing, and repair foods. They sound like great lists don't they? I pulled all my information together and got out my biggest notepad, convinced I would need every page to collate such a list, then realized something.

Superfoods, instant energy foods, endurance, strengthening and healing foods are the same foods. Isn't that great? Not a whole great book of lists to stock your kitchen with and figure out how to use. Just a handful of vegetables, fruits, nuts, seeds, fats, protein and you have it all. All you need for fuel, medicine and super health and vitality.

Food as Medicine

As Hippocrates said way back, "Let food be thy medicine and medicine be thy food."

One of the reasons to eat a varied diet is it provides a well-rounded supply of all we need to remain healthy. If we do become sick, we can use it as medicine as well as fuel as this wise man said.

Research has shown chicken soup really does help us recover from colds. Spirulina provides the building blocks of life and numerous minerals; the root kudzu soothes the gut and supports the immune system while vegetables and fruits burst with energy and antioxidants to neutralize inflammation.

Rich bone broth fortifies our defenses, flooding our body with super nutrition and fermented foods feed our all important gut bacteria, making sure we can break down our food and absorb the nutrients that are released. Chamomile and rooibos tea soothes our nerves, herbs tackle infections, and vegetables and fruits help keep our immune systems in top working order.

All animals, including us, instinctively know what we need to eat, for fuel, for medicine, for pleasure. We have known these things since the dawn of time, but since the advent of miracle drugs, we seem to have forgotten this. Part of bringing your life back to a whole is changing your idea about food and becoming reacquainted with its purpose.

Giving our bodies what they need allows real healing to begin. Already, we see that with food as the fuel that powers our lives and as soothing medicine, what we should eat becomes simple. If we further develop the ability to listen to our body and what it may need, healing can happen at a rapid pace.

Recently I had the opportunity to test this theory again, as if the last decade wasn't enough! A trained and experienced health and wellness health coach I may be, but I am no more immune to reckless diet and life choices than the next person. If there is a difference between you and me, it is perhaps in my knowledge of what to do to repair the damage and get myself back on my feet quickly.

Having pushed my body way beyond its limits, it protested by putting me back on the couch in the disguise of a viral infection. It was a pretty good one too. A feeling hit by a truck, swollen glands, night sweats, can't stand up without wanting to pass out kind of viral infection that would have poleaxed me prior to my journey from couch to life.

My treatment?

This is what I ate for three or four days:
3lbs Broccoli
2lbs Cauliflower
4 Cups Kale
4 Cups Fresh Tomatoes

4 Avocados
4lbs Strawberries
4 Oranges
Coconut Oil
Raw Cacao
Water
Chamomile Tea
Rooibos Tea

This time I did need the intervention of antiviral medication as well, but what would have kept me on the couch for months took away just three workdays. There is no recovery time needed either. I am recovered, strong, healthy and a little wiser, until the next time anyway!

I had another great list I was going to share with you, all about the diseases and conditions each fruit and vegetable can protect against. It was two pages with six columns on each page with an impressive list of health benefits. I found myself drawn into looking at the best food to treat this and that, then realized something.

Less than a dozen vegetables and fruits, all from this continent, a handful of nuts and seeds and a few cups of tea can help protect you from heart disease, aid digestion, improve lung capacity, cushion your joints, protect against Alzheimer's disease, stabilize blood pressure and blood sugar, boost your memory, lift your mood, calm your stressed nerves, strengthen bones, support the immune system, banish bruises, protect against cancer, stokes, high cholesterol and heart disease, enhance blood flow, aid in weight loss, quiet a cold, sooth sore throats, kill bacteria, funguses, viruses and put an end to insomnia.

Still hate your veggies?

Finding Your Optimal Diet for Recovery
Removing first gluten, then dairy, then all grains from my diet proved to be the answer for me. It was shocking for me to realize the food I had grown up

eating was actually making me sick to the point of needing those all important infusions of other peoples' immune systems to function. It was even harder to comprehend these foods were responsible for reducing my life to the couch watching the Lifetime Movie Network.

It wasn't just the foods I was eating that had put me there. It was what I wasn't eating that had just as much of an impact. Years of insufficient nutrition coupled with a high stress lifestyle and the baggage of almost half a century on this earth.

I tell you this so you can keep an open mind about what the underlying causes of your illness could be. On reflection, I can see how issues with these foods have in fact shown up all my life. Watching the gradual decline of my health over a life of eating things my body could not handle, I now wonder, not that these foods make me sick; but that my miraculous, tenacious little body continued on even after so much abuse. It has to be said I was not looking good, but how I survived is a complete miracle!

My optimal diet for *recovery* turned out to be one free from grains and dairy, packed with vegetables, fruit, seeds, nuts, good fats, some carefully selected super foods and a little high quality animal protein. It has many names; Primal Diet, modified Paleo; I call it Sue's diet!

The foods I select each day and the combinations I eat them in is determined by how I'm feeling and what I want to do with my day. This is what provides the variety in my diet. If I have a very busy week, I can live happily on my Super Green Smoothie's and baked vegetables during the day, knowing not only are my bases are covered, I have plenty of fuel to power through my day.

A bowl of pumpkin and sunflower seeds with a few raisins and some energy balls to munch on and I've added nutrient packed snacks to my super food smoothies and nutrient dense veggies. Top class nutrition all day without the need to stop, cook or clean. Neither do I have to deal with the side effects of food that really isn't.

A side of top quality animal protein on a pile of vegetables and a delicious, nutritious dessert at the end of my busy day and my nourishment, fuel and medicinal needs are met. If I'm stressed, fatigued or unwell, I reach for nutrient dense, easy to absorb foods, things like soups, smoothies and the ubiquitous veggies. More than anything else, these are my go to foods for healing, repair and energy. Nuts and seeds give me staying power and endurance long after I've eaten them. Roots, fruits and brassicas[8]* with a few nuts and seeds, and a side of humanely raised, organic pastured animal protein, that's me.

Notice it is all whole food, as nature makes it.

How do you find *your* optimal diet for recovery?

I did it by trial and error and it took me years. There were many wrong turns along the way and so many times I felt I was stumbling blindly on, which in truth I was. I played with a lot of foods, some which worked, some that tasted so bad I couldn't care less what they could cure and some which made me feel even worse, though I didn't think that was possible!

We are all wonderfully unique and what works for one person does not work for another. We have different genetic and cultural backgrounds, live in numerous different environmental conditions and those are just the most obvious variables.

One man's food is another man's poison, so listening to outdated, mainstream advice about what to eat will not help you. Neither will wading through the masses of information available about food. All profess to have *the* answer, which could only be true if there were such a thing as *the* human being. But there isn't. There are human beings plural, in all their glorious, wonderful variety!

There is a way through; I found it myself, though it took me an agonizingly long time. Enrolling in the Institute for Integrative Nutrition® accelerated my journey and helped me combine my own knowledge and experience with the science that lay behind what I had done and why it had worked.

The selection of recipes at the end of this book is a great place to start. Free from the most common foods that cause allergies and food intolerances, a few simple changes can add nutrient dense foods that will make you

8   * Brassicas are the cruciferous vegetables like cabbages, Brussels sprouts and broccoli that provide high amounts of vitamin C, soluble fiber and multiple nutrients with potent anti cancer properties.

feel a whole lot better. If you join me on my website, you'll be able to access tons of really cool tools to help accelerate your journey. There you can connect with others, take classes, sign up for coaching and workshops and lose yourself in the reference library or online recipe books.

Explore links to diets for specific health conditions and take a look at my "Mix and Match Plan," for eating a whole foods diet in about the same time it would take you to put your shoes on, grab your keys and drive to the nearest fast food drive through each day. Forty two servings of vegetables, twenty one of fruits, thirteen recipes, three delicious, nutritious meals a day for seven days with about two hours of work in your kitchen.

Take the challenge and set a goal for the amount of vegetables and fruit you want to eat. Do you want to start with the basics, or is repairing, replacing and rejuvenating your worn out body your goal? Perhaps you want to experience super energy, or better yet, you may be so inspired by now, you want it all. I know I did!

CHAPTER 7

The Mind Body Connection

The ability of the mind to cause disease seems to be where we go when someone fails to recover from illness within a certain period of time. If we remain sick after recovery should have happened, well there must be some deficiency or default in thinking that keeps us sick.

This attitude used to drive me insane when I was stuck on the couch. The idea that I, with all the effort I had put into life despite been too sick to live it, was being told it was that very same thinking that made me sick was too much. That if I could just "pull myself together," I could get better if I really wanted to. Just typing these words makes my stomach tighten and the feelings of injustice and the indignity they rightly provoked is threatening to overwhelm me, so I'll move on.

Many well-meaning medical professionals have told us our answers are in our minds, but I want to make this crystal clear. That is true for all of us about every single thing in our lives. What no one tells you is exactly how you are supposed to change your mind to change your body. It is no easy thing to do when you have no idea how to do it or where to start.

The food we eat directly affects the chemicals our bodies make which in turn affects our mood, our thinking, our emotional landscape. That piece of broccoli you eat doesn't just contain vitamins, minerals and fiber. It contains information, exchanged at a cellular level that allows us to make all we need to keep this amazing bio-computer of a body running in tip-top shape. When we run smoothly, who doesn't feel happy?

For those of us who have been chronically sick, exhaustion is a major part of our daily experience. Getting through our days is challenging enough at the best of times, so even if we *did* know how to do it, where, oh where, would we find the energy?

This is why I began this journey by creating more energy. Before you can do anything, you have to have something to work with. Creating energy allows us to take steps to improve the strength in our body that in turn gives us the strength we need to start looking at other areas of our lives that may be contributing to our continued malaise. Notice I say contribute, not cause!

You have been following along though and having earned some great energy points, you have something to play with. So where do you start?

Most advice would have you looking to your thoughts, why they got there, dragging them out of the toilet so to speak, and thinking of affirmations to negate them and replacing them with happy thoughts. I say this tongue in cheek. These techniques do work, but again, it is the cart before the horse.

Starting at this place puts all your energy and action in one section of your life. Though your mind may feel better with this exercise, the body still has not received what it needs to begin the repair and with no energy to do anything, the knowing can be a devastating tease!

There is a mind body connection. They cannot be separated. What happens in the mind affects the body and what happens on, in and to the body affects the mind.

Where things get really confusing is when the medical profession has us believing our illness is a fabrication of our mind. This happens when all the tools doctors have at their disposal have been thrown at us and have failed to return an answer.

So where do you start? Put nutrition front and center of your life. Improve your nutrition, start seeing and using food as fuel and as medicine and the increase in energy you experience will change your thoughts. All those wonderful nutrients coursing through your veins jump off the super highway of lifeblood wherever needed to nourish, to repair, and to replenish your body. Who couldn't help feeling more positive in this enriching environment?

Your thoughts are happier because your body now has the materials it needs to make the hormones required to run this miracle called your body. Your brain is bathed in all the elements it needs and surrounded by so much food; it would take a determined and persistent effort to remain grumpy with such abundance of goodness!

Now you're in the right frame of mind and have what you need to start looking at where changes in your thinking could make your journey to health much faster. Lets face it; being stuck on the couch is not for the faint of heart. To be there, some negative thinking inevitably crept into your mind and took up camp. A spring-cleaning is in order and with energy under your belt, you can move forward in leaps and bounds.

Though I have talked about the nutritious food we eat, I want to quickly point out how bringing life back to the whole works time and time again, in any area of your life.

Nutrition is in the center because it is required for all the area of your life to function. When I talk about nutrition though, I mean way more than the food we eat, even though that is where we put most of our attention.

Here's a great example.

You realize your diet has been deficient in some vital essentials for a long time and wisely decide to incorporate the mighty kale in your diet in as many ways as possible. The addition of these nutrients feels like being infused with the elixir of life! Your body is beginning to feel different, like you might actually be able to move from where you have been stuck for so long.

What you may not appreciate is the other ways you have nourished yourself and the impact it has on all areas of your life. You have taken a time out to see where you are and made a conscious decision to somehow move forward. You have taken action by eating more kale and this act of loving care is maybe the first time you've been nice to yourself for a very long time.

Your mind is soothed and your spirit soars as you see, not dysfunction and disease, but courage, determination and dare I say strength. Yes strength. The one thing you feel you have been missing all this time turns out to be one of the things that has carried you through your ordeal to the threshold of recovery. How about that!

How many parts of you might be nourished by this revelation?

We'll talk more about nourishing yourself with things other than food in the next chapter, but see how much power just adding something like kale has to your diet has? If this can happen with kale, what might happen if you start to throw around some super foods as well?

Integrating Food with Life for Optimal Health and Performance

As we've seen, nourishing ourselves with food impacts not just our body, but also all aspects of our lives. If it has the power to do that, what might happen if we consciously used food to enhance these different aspects?

Nature, in her infinite wisdom, has made it easy for us to know which foods we need to eat by making them look like the part of the body that benefits the most when we eat them.

A great example of this is cauliflower. When you look at it, what does it remind you of? And guess what? It *is* a super food for your brain. Leafy greens like kale look a lot like your lungs, covered with vessels to transport oxygen rich blood to the rest of your body. Not surprising then that they are super foods for the lungs. Blueberries, one of the highest food sources of antioxidants, are packed with nutritious vitamins and minerals that are particularly beneficial to the eyes. Looking at them end on, you can see the resemblance.

Books have been written about the subject and it is the area of much research that I find fascinating. You now know enough about it to start making different choices about the food you eat. Next time you're in the fruit and vegetable aisle of the supermarket, look at each fruit and vegetable and try to determine which part of the body it will most benefit. I guarantee you'll never look at food the same way again!

Lets take this analogy with food a little further.

We established the mind body connection and now understand that the two are inextricably linked. What happens to the body affects the mind and what happens to the mind affects the body. We have seen how food affects our mood and how we can change our mood by changing the foods we eat.

We've covered the mind and body that drive our lives, but what of our soul? How can a plate of vegetables nourish your soul?

We are all familiar with the humble potato. A whole civilization all but perished when it disappeared from their diet. Buried deep in the ground, it is the root that stores and releases nutrients to nourish the potato plant which grows above ground.

There is a whole family called root vegetables and as you would expect, they all live underground and are the nutrient keepers and providers for the plants they sustain above ground.

The foods we eat provide not just overall nourishment for our body, but nourishment for specific areas, so think for a minute about the root vegetable. Rooting its plant to the earth, it stores all the nutrients the plant needs to thrive and flourish. Everything it needs is contained in that root and there are even reserves available should the environment turn hostile.

I mentioned earlier how I use food to power my day, selecting what I need to accomplish all the things I want to do. To power through a busy day without feeling like a wrung out dish rag at the end of it requires super nutrition, full of energy. As the day comes to a close, it 's time to shut some of that energy down, time to connect to something else, time to relax and rejuvenate and restore. This is absolutely not the time to be eating high energy foods.

A delicious dish of roasted root vegetables, for example will release its nutrition to you over time, gradually yielding those all important rejuvenating ingredients as you plug yourself back into earth and recharge. Sprinkled with fresh herbs that recharge your immune system and taking minutes to prepare, who would not find themselves craving such a meal? Sure convenience food may sound good, and may even taste good, but does it ground you to the earth? Does it center you and make you whole? Does it provide sustained nutrition over hours to rejuvenate your body?

Will you ever look at food the same way again?

I sincerely hope not! I'll talk more about learning to listen to your body in a minute, but the next time you have a yen for a particular food, pay attention. Your body is giving you an enormous clue!

With all this talk about using specific foods to nourish specific areas of our bodies, I want to say again that it isn't really possible to separate ourselves, focus on the parts and experience good, long lasting health. I want to close this part by saying there is no such thing as a food for this or a food for that. That thinking lives in the land of separation.

There is just food, all of which nourishes us to one degree or another. By focusing on the food we eat and making different decisions about what we put in our mouths, we nourish ourselves in so many ways. Who could compute the nutritional value of providing quality food, taking the time to listen to their body to select exactly what it needs to be its best? The love, care and attention that displays nourishes us at a deep, deep level, perhaps much more than the nutritional profile of the food we eat, affecting all areas of our lives.

Everything In Balance Not Moderation

How many times have we heard the statement, "all things in moderation?" What does that mean exactly? What is one mans moderation could well be another's death sentence, so how do we know the right degree of "moderate," for us?

What happens if we do things that are bad for us, in moderation?

Great questions, though I think it is an enormous diversion to try and answer them. I think moderation is really about giving ourselves permission to do something we know we shouldn't do, without guilt.

It is a great responsibility being a human being, so letting off steam every once in a while by eating that burger in defiance can be a liberating act! That said; there are some things that are not just bad for us but will kill us stone dead, so even a moderate intake is unadvisable.

Suppose we were to reword that statement by saying "everything in balance," instead? Would that make a difference?

You may have followed all the advice in this book and found yourself spending considerable time off the couch. You now know how food powers your life and are used to selecting your food based on your day rather than what the latest television commercial is telling you to eat.

You've had a busy week and have energized yourself with kale and super green smoothies each day. To bring yourself down in the evening so you can sleep, you eat a generous plate of root vegetables roasted in coconut oil and sprinkled with herbs. You have worked non-stop through the week. It's Friday and not only are you standing, you're in pretty good shape.

Does that look or sound like balance to you?

As you read those words, did you hear a little voice saying, "what about this and that, how is that balance?"

I don't believe a balanced diet is about eating a particular selection of foods day in and day out to make sure our nutritional profiles are met one hundred percent every day. First of all, how would we determine the optimum nutritional profile for a human day so you could make sure all your bases were covered? It depends on so much; activity level, stress levels, you'd have to calculate it every day to make sure you had everything you need.

No. I believe balance is about providing ourselves with what we need when we need it based on our lives and what we want to live them. No wonder none of us has been able to find balance in our lives up to this point. What we thought was balance, turned out to be regimented, unyielding compliance to an ideal diet for *the* human that doesn't exist. We do exist. In all our unique, complex variety!

This opens the door for us to be bad without guilt. When we know for the most part we have a healthy, balanced diet and lifestyle, indulging in something not so good for us becomes enormous fun; a deviation from an otherwise adherent, sensible life and it feels wonderfully liberating!

Just imagine how freeing such a life would be. How much more could you do with your life if you ate for performance, fuel and medicine? You would select food for its ability to help you live your life and do all the things you want, with ample room for deviation and fun. Is that a diet and lifestyle you think you may be able to adopt for the rest of your life?

A Connection To Something Bigger

Having had our lives, as we know them taken away by chronic illness, it has been easy to separate ourselves from just about everything. Unable to play like others, we felt disconnected from all those around us who could. The financial impact of our illness has left our bank accounts empty, often with enormous debt as we have struggled to find answers.

Feeling adrift and unconnected to anything was often one of the most scary and difficult things to deal with about my illness. Feeling so far removed from everyone is a crushingly lonely experience, but I don't have to tell you that.

I had faith and belief, but without the ability to express that in my world, I felt stunted, confined and trapped way beyond the bonds of my physical body. I yearned to feel connected to something, anything. I really, really wanted to find a way to start playing again.

This urge we all have to connect with something larger than ourselves is not often talked about. Not being able to contribute to this great experiment called life has a devastating effect on our bodies and minds.

Whether it is a connection to a person, our community, our planet, nature, what many of us call God in all the wonderful names it is described; it is an integral part of what it means to be human. It is the essence of who we are and to lose sight of it casts us adrift in a sea of disconnection, loneliness and despair. Rare is the human who can walk their lives without the need of others.

Starved of this connection, once I had used the energy I had created to begin my journey to health, my next mission was to reconnect with life. I needed to start getting myself out into the world, to see how I might play with everyone else. I remember this being a key turning point in my recovery; so lets see what reconnecting and discovering a purpose can do to accelerate your journey.

All the broccoli in the entire world cannot save you from a life of loneliness, disconnection and feeling unfulfilled. It's powerful stuff, a super food, even with amazing cancer fighting properties, but it doesn't have the power to do that. Who would want an optimally nourished body if they felt alone with no one to share their life with? Would such a person even care how they looked?

Reconnecting is a very powerful step and I warn you now, once taken, there may be no turning back. Starting with baby steps, I dipped my toes in the water of my community and I'm still trying to recover from the response. If you can find a way to connect with your community and are willing to show up to help others, strap yourself in because your life is about to take off!

We've come a long way in these pages. Having been stuck on the couch for so long, many of us believed we would never be able to get up and participate in life again. Having created energy, we have put it to use in healing our broken bodies and spirits and now we understand we have control over our health. We are confident we can actually start contemplating a life permanently off the couch. In all the time of your confinement, your energy has been spent in somehow surviving your devastating circumstances, so this is a new lease on life.

We disconnected from ourselves, our lives that could only exist in our minds up to this point, often our families, our communities and the very world we live in. Its time to reconnect so we can take things to the next level.

CHAPTER 8

Life Beyond Chronic Illness

The Bigger Picture – Purpose and Service

Like me, you may never have believed you would get to this point in your life where you could consider the bigger questions of just why you might be on this earth and what you want to do while you are here. Perhaps before you became sick, the chances that you'd stop to ponder such things was slim to none. I used to joke that I didn't stop long enough to notice there *were* roses, much less smell them!

But here you are. You've had the wind knocked out of your sails, your life as you knew it taken away and you have found a way to pick yourself up again. How incredible are you!

So what will you do with all your newfound energy?

As I whiled away the hours on my couch, I made a promise, no, I swore, that if I ever found a way to get myself back up again, I would find a way to help others who wanted to do the same. Sounds ridiculous that the mind conceives such things when there is no logical sense it will ever be possible, but there it is.

As my strength returned, I found myself involved in a different project, one that would lead me, through some beautiful twists and turns of life right to where I am now, typing these words to you in the hope they will help get you *"From Couch to Life!"*

I wanted to build a website where all the local artists and crafters could advertise their beautiful items for sale with a percentage of each sale going to a local non-profit of the buyer's choice. Called Eastern Sierra Crafts, I had contacted many artists who were interested and I wanted to take the business to the next level. When I was invited to give a talk at a Rotary meeting, I knew it was the perfect opportunity.

I had no idea when I walked into that first lunch meeting in 2011 that my life was about to change forever. As I sit writing this on New Year's Eve, 2014, Eastern Sierra Crafts still lives in its three ring binder and for now, that is where it will have to remain. I have big plans for it in the future!

What happened after I was invited to join the Rotary Club of Bishop can only be described as a fairy tale. I still remember the email I sent to then President, Mike Gable, letting him know that I could probably guarantee my attendance at two of the four monthly meetings and I would do my best to participate in as many service projects in my community as possible, but my first priority was my marriage.

I'm still not really sure what I meant by that, except the daily rituals of everyday life were exhausting, leaving little or no energy for anything else. But a strange thing started to happen. As I used my energy to begin serving others, first cooking in the soup kitchen, then creating and running programs in the Elementary School, I began to notice that although I didn't feel any better, I was able to do so much more. There were still no guarantees I would be able to get off the couch consistently, but as I made the commitments, I somehow found a way to meet them.

It didn't always work and often, my sometimes reckless pushing would incapacitate me for weeks, but being asked to play with a group of Rotarians turned out to be just what I needed. No medicine in the world could have done for me what those wonderful people did and still do for me! Knowing my back was covered if I couldn't make an event took all the pressure off for me. If I woke in the morning and knew not only wasn't it a driving day, I was going to be cemented to the couch, someone else would and could step in.

Except one night when I was preparing to present Ms. Hammie's 3rd Grade class with their own personally dedicated Thesauruses to take home.

All twenty seven books were spread out on my dining room table and all twenty seven books needed personal labels printed and stuck in the front cover.

That morning, I knew I was in trouble. I couldn't stand upright without wanting to pass out and waves of nausea kept me rushing to the bathroom. Bathed in sweat, the day was drawing to a close and still the books remained untouched. I called around. No one was available. I started to panic and tears flowed down my cheeks. I remember feeling an utter failure, the frustration and anger overwhelming me.

I suddenly looked down and realized what I was doing. Having started reading circles with Ms. Hamilton, Bishop Rotarians had been going to the school to read with the students; seven Rotarians every week for the whole school year. I wanted to celebrate the end of the year by buying each student their own thesaurus, so I asked the club to approve the expense, and here they were, spread all over my dining table.

There I was, about to give 27 children a gift of a book, dedicated to them. Some of them didn't have the luxury of owning their own books, so this was going to be a big deal. The tears dried and the biggest smile appeared on my face as I realized the gift *I* had been given.

I'm not going to lie and say I found the energy to zip through the task, I didn't. It took me hour after painful hour and I had to sit down many, many times. But I did it. I can't begin to explain what it did for me the next day when I made it through the doors of the school, bundled up with books to give away. Food for the soul, food for the mind; not even the mighty kale can compete with that kind of nutrition!

Having seen how far this had taken me from my couch, the next year found me launching another program in the school. I'd received a newsletter from my local bank telling me they were teaching financial literacy to 12th graders and I thought it would make a brilliant addition to our Rotary Club's literacy outreach. Approaching the school, myself and another Rotarian, Josh Ingram, suggested starting with the 5th grade. They agreed and asked us to teach it to all four classes, approximately one hundred and thirty students. Seriously? Yes, they were, very!

Though there were no dramatic moments like the thesauruses had presented me with, I found myself embarking on a journey that challenged my brain-fogged mind to its limits. Dissecting the www.myclassroomeconmy.org program and working out how to introduce it to so many students over a whole school year exhausted me physically and mentally. As I was fond of saying, my mood remained in the toilet much of the time as I struggled to get my brain to engage. Month after month, I worked tirelessly to pull everything together, spending more than one hundred hours on the project.

Finally it was launch day and I still remember the immense control it took to corral my thoughts so I could teach a class. I thought seeing the program unfold without a hitch and the students completely engage with it was enough to keep me smiling for the rest of my life, but in one of those beautiful synchronicities in life, I was about to be presented with something that knocked my socks off.

The Rotary District our club belongs to, District 5190, give awards each year for many things and unknown to me, I was nominated for one. The District Governor came to town and summoned me up to the podium to be presented with, wait for it, an Energizer Award!

Yes you read that right, an Energizer Award! Me, the stuck on the couch, struggling and swearing my way though impossible days of frustration was in fact an energizer. Never mind smiling for the rest of my life, it is two years later and I still burst out laughing when I think about that! Here's what is printed on my certificate that has pride of place in my office:

"Presented in recognition of your special energy, vitality and spirit to positively impact your club, community and the world with your dedication and commitment to the object of Rotary. The energizer emblem symbolizes the structure of a carbon atom, the basis of all life."

Me, with energy and vitality. I will treasure that moment for the rest of my life. The moment I realized that stuck on the couch I may have been, but here I stood, proud and tall, an Energizer!

We often hear that people who live a life of service have a longer life expectancy than others and for the longest time, I wondered why that might be. These experiences showed me exactly why.

What on the surface looks like me donating time to others in a terrific altruistic outreach is in fact me taking advantage of the opportunity to re-engage my mind, dust off some seriously rusty skills and test the water to see just what I *could* accomplish. I distinctly remember the decision to "use" Rotary to test and push the limit of my abilities, and before long, it had become almost a full time job.

What did I get back? The chance to hone my skills and use them to write this book, launch an online wellness community to help others recover their health and the discovery that far from my life being over, it has in so many ways, only just begun.

When we do show up in service to others, when we put ourselves and our own needs aside and devote ourselves to a larger idea than us, we find that as fast as we give, more is received. It opens a door to a whole new world; of opportunities, of possibilities and before long, it becomes impossible to distinguish who is the giver and who the receiver. This is what I call the experience of being in the flow of life, with all the energy and vitality you would expect from such an experience.

Now you have retrieved some of your precious energy, start giving some away and see if it doesn't come back multiplied! Just as food provides super health for your body, this expanded view is rocket fuel for your life's dreams and desires.

Finding Your Passion

Most people take their ideas and dreams to the graves with them and I thought I was destined to be one of them. Getting through a day was hard enough, figuring out I may have a passion much less what it could be or what I could do with it was not on my radar. Yet like many of us, there was this nagging feeling in the back of my mind, an empty feeling in the pit of my stomach as I contemplated my life amounting to nothing more than being a bump on the log or life, or should I say couch.

It was this very urge, squashed somewhere deep inside that woke me in the night feeling anxious and panicky. It was this urge that kept me restless, on edge, propelling me to find the answer, not to the source of my disease and cure, but an answer of how to live life in spite of it.

Aware time was ticking by in a haze of pain and despair as I had written in 2010, I realized it was futile spending any more time researching my condition for answers. That road had taken me to meet some of the most beautiful souls, so I'm not going to call it a detour. One thing I learned about putting all my focus on my condition. It got bigger and bigger, as everything we give focus and attention to does.

Before I knew it, my whole life was consumed by my illness. It consumed my thoughts, my speech, and my time. It was my life. I lived and breathed it. So much precious energy and I became sicker and sicker.

It seems ironic that I am finishing this book on New Years Eve, 2014, when my journey from couch to life began in earnest on New Year's Eve, 2009. Sick of being sick and living a life of sickness, I made one resolution that year; just one.

"2010 is going to be the best year ever despite my illness and whether I get better or not."

That was it. Just that handful of words. With no idea how it was going to happen or what was going to happen, just an unequivocal statement backed up by unwavering belief that it was so.

Five years later, I am off my couch and haven't had to spend one day there for over a year, involuntarily anyway. In the last five years, I have accomplished more than I could imagine possible in my wildest of dreams. I am continually blessed with opportunities to serve and the more I do, the more comes back to me. Finding my passion was the rocket fuel that propelled my life forward. So many times I have to stop myself to realize this really has happened and I'm not stuck in some dream.

How might you begin to find your passion to propel your health forward?

I could have started every single chapter and bullet point in this book with the words, "Give yourself the biggest gift of your life and find a health and wellness coach," though that may have been overkill. I can't stress enough how much they can help you uncover things just like this. They can help you do in months what can take years of trial and error to figure out on your own.

Join me at the From Couch To Life! Website where you'll find many tools to help you uncover your passion. Could it be that you want to use all that you have learned from your own journey to help other on theirs? If so, perhaps you are also a health and wellness coach health and wellness coach with an important message to share with others.

Be The Change; You Are The Solution to 21st Century Problems

One of the reasons you are reading this book is you or someone you know has been devastated by a chronic illness and is confined to the couch. With more than fifty percent of us suffering from chronic disease, it would be hard not to be aware of it. It fills our newspapers and airwaves, consumes hours of debate as we ponder how to reduce the horrendous financial and other burdens for this percentage of the population.

We live in very sobering times. Our planet isn't in much better shape than most of us. Global temperatures are rising; pollution fills the earth, our homes, and our lives. Increasing numbers of people need to be fed; yet the food available leaves even those in prosperous countries malnourished and starving, rattling around inside ever increasing frames.

Our children suffer from record amounts of disease, many unable to concentrate and focus at school, the effects of which are life long. Water is running low and the economy is not balanced and conducive to a happy healthy life for all.

Many things have to change and it is going to take all of us to make that change. Gandhi said, "Be the change you wish to see," and I love that quote. It speaks to every one of us individually to do something about the things around us we don't like and don't want to see any more.

You have just undertaken an incredible journey and against all odds, managed to rise from your couch. Though others told you all you needed was to pull yourself up by your bootstraps, they never imagined you would or could, yet here you stand, yes stand. Victorious. Triumphant.

I have mentioned throughout his book the courage, tenacity, the shear focus and determination it has taken you to come this far. So many don't even attempt the journey, so realize what a true hero you are. These skills are not to be taken lightly. They are precisely the kind of skills this world needs to tackle some of these problems.

Were will you start to make a difference?

Do you feel called to help others do what you have just done?

Are you passionate about the health of children in our communities?

What is it that makes you hurt, that makes you sad, that makes you want to make a difference? What do you think might happen to you, your community, to this country and this world if you were to take what you have learned and apply it to such a problem? Perhaps we'll find ourselves working in solutions instead of being stuck in discussions about what is wrong and who is to blame.

Now you have your freedom again, what burning issues do you want to change? How will you make a difference and be the change in your community?

An Important Note About Recovery

Whether you believe it or not, you have already taken the all-important first step by reading this book. I'm not saying it is so packed with age-old truths and never before revealed wisdoms, that you have been instantly cured. That would be silly. You can't deny though that I have given you a few things to think about.

The very fact that I have given you a different way to think about your life, your food, your lifestyle; means your outlook has already changed. Even if my words have cemented your belief that you are destined to spend the rest of your life on the couch, I'm pretty confident you look at your life differently now.

When I talk about going from couch to life, I want to make something very clear. I refer to the couch not just as a physical thing and place, but a frame of mind, a state of being. For some people, however much they change their beliefs, attitudes, diets, whatever is possible to change to live their best life possible, they will remain within the confines of that couch.

On the couch or on your feet, top quality food for the body and mind is crucial; so don't be tempted to think making any kind of change is not worth the effort if you find you are in this category. In fact, I would go so far as to say top quality nutrition of every kind is more important for you than anything else. A life on the couch comes with many challenges, and deconditioning is one of them. Over time, that in itself, can lead to further health issues that you just don't need to deal with.

I also ask you to consider if it's possible to escape even while you are cemented and bound to it. Could a change of mind, of attitude, of the way you see your point and purpose in life take your mind so far away from its chains, the fact your body remains there hardly matter?

The idea there are those who keep the high watch so to speak, fills me with gratitude. Not distracted by the everyday "doings," your contribution is perhaps greater. Making sure that despite all your daily struggles, you find a way to contribute to all the good, positive thoughts in your community, acting like an invisible energy field and lifting us all. If that describes you, I thank you with all my heart.

I believe every single life matters. Every expression of life is important. Every one of us has a purpose and unique talents to offer the world. Everyone. Without exception. We all have opportunities and challenges in life, regardless of physical circumstance, so though not all will physically rise from the couch, all can soar above it in every other way imaginable.

CHAPTER 9

The One Page Life

Your Life Simplified

Writing this book feels like I've been on my journey all over again. I've been looking forward to getting to this point, not because it's the end of this part of the journey and this book, but because, now I am here and have coalesced all I have learned into these pages, I can stop, take a breath and appreciate how far I have come and all I have achieved.

If anyone had asked me five years ago if I could have done half the things I have, because I embarked on this journey, I would have laughed so hard; I would have fallen off my couch. You can imagine I have learned much along the way and I want to share one of those precious gems here; *"The One Page Life."*

By now, you should be used to being able to create energy at will using all the techniques you have learned in this book. You have done some incredible things with your newfound life off the couch and are continuing to make some great changes.

Is it possible to take things to the next level and achieve more?

Yes!

I guess it was a reaction to the masses and masses of information I've had to wade through to decipher the pearls of wisdom necessary to return to health. That and the wonderful training I have received at the Institute for Integrative Nutrition®. When I signed up at the end of 2013, to study nutrition, I had no idea I'd be finishing the year as a health and wellness coach and author of this book!

Even with all the energy in the world, it is no easy thing to become a certified health and wellness coach in less than one year while also writing a book and donating hundreds of volunteer hours to my community. It took master planning and execution. Necessity being the mother of invention, I devised what I call, "The One Page Life."

The basis of "The One Page Life," is if what you are trying to do does not fit on one page, it is way too complicated!

You would be amazed at the clarity this seemingly simple exercise creates.

Everything and I mean everything I do has fit on one page.

A marketing plan for my business? One page. My weekly schedule incorporating clients, studying, service, writing? One page. How to write this book? One page.

In fact, it was the one page approach that allowed me to write this in less than a week. For sure, I have been burning the midnight oil, but a book, in six days, how is that even possible?

"The One Page Life," is how!

To show you how this works, lets take the entire contents of this book and condense it down to one page. Why in the world would you want to write 25,000 words, and then condense them down to one page you might ask, but bear with me here?

There is of course a ton of information that lies behind the one page of anything. The point of the one page is to have you laser focus on what you want to achieve and put that front and center of everything you do.

Once your focus is clear and written down on one page, it becomes your blueprint for everything else that needs to happen. If you find yourself straying to page two, you have made it too complicated and it will not be easily accomplished. So here it goes; 25,000 words into one page!

Prescription for Health

Prescribed By: From Couch to Life!

Read This Book

Install New Software; Recovery Is Possible

Clean Up Your Diet

Create More Energy

Detox Your Life

Design Your Optimal Diet

Integrate Body Mind and Soul Food

Implement "The One Page Life"

Employ a Health and Wellness Coach

Be The Change / Live Your Passion

** Warning **

* Do not exceed 3 Actions Per Step
* Significant increases in energy will be noticeable and will intensify with each additional step taken
*Stopping this prescription before finished will result in incomplete transition from couch to life

Signed: _____   Date: _____
Sue Lyndes - Health and Wellness Coach

Create *Your* One Page Life

Though this one technique alone will free up untold amounts of energy, it didn't make any sense to include it in the section on creating energy. That was way back at the beginning of the book when the goal was to create energy to begin your journey to health. Who could care about a "One Page Life," then?

You have come a long way since then and now is the time for you to start designing your own one page life. You can start with your whole life or choose one area and write a "One Page Action Plan" to begin moving from where you are to where you want to be.

Now all you have to do is pick a starting point and begin. That's it. When you find questions coming up, go back to your plan. If you're tempted to expand things but spill over into page two, it's too complicated. Go back to your one page plan; it's all you need.

Now imagine what could happen if you took the area you were working on and placed it in the center of your life as you did in Chapter Three in Bringing Your Life Back To A Whole?" These two things, one focusing on what you need, the other a one page outline of how you are going to get there will take you to a whole new level of achievement and performance.

Of course, having got control of your life, you might decide to spend some time contemplating which of life's challenges you could use your unique talents to help fix.

Just not on the couch. In fact, why don't you throw that old thing out!

CHAPTER 10

Healthy Foods And Delicious Recipes

n this last chapter, you'll find some great information on healthy, energy packed, healing foods. Take a look and see how easy it is to make delicious, nutritious foods.

Next, look through the selection of recipes and see how my "Mix and Match" approach to dinners will take about three hours to produce and will provide you with twenty one meals, twelve snacks, six desserts, thirty six servings of vegetables and seventeen servings of superfoods.

Just The Basics – Easy Total Nutrition Recipes

I have included a selection of what I call "Just the Basics," recipes for dishes that form the basis of my everyday diet. Once prepared, they can be mixed and matched in multiple combinations to provide delicious, nutritious meals in minutes. With that many doses of super fuel and medicine, your body should find it impossible to remain sick.

All the recipes I share in this section do quadruple duty and can be used for breakfast, lunch, dessert, or snacks. Nearly all of them anyway, delicious as fruit is, I didn't count it as a lunch. Roast broccoli with sesame seeds didn't make it into the desserts category either, but you get the idea. The combinations you come up with and the few simple additions you add to optimize a meal plan for your life will provide you with all the variety you need.

Each batch of a recipe provides four generous servings with the exception of the smoothie recipe that provides two.

At www.fromcouchtolife.com, you'll find fifty recipes that you can use to start designing your own seven-day meal plan. You'll also find a blank "Seven Day Meal Plan" document that you can print and use to keep track of your favorites.

When designed your own meal plan, it's worth considering that the average person tends to cycle through just seven different meals a week. If you think about it, how many different dishes do you make each week?

Keeping it simple makes it much easier to stick to a diet that makes health and vitality your default. The meal combinations show you how you can eat thirty six servings of vegetables and seventeen of super foods every week. Don't be intimidated by this number. I promise you, it is way easier than you think and totally delicious as well as nutritious.

Before you plunge headlong into a diet overhaul, consider this cautionary note.

You will have read this at the beginning of this book, but it bears repeating here. We often think that because something is a whole food and hopefully organic, consuming it can only be good for us. As we discussed in Chapter Five, that is not always the case. What works for one person does not necessarily work for another and one person's food is another person's poison, so it is important you check with your physician before you make radical changes to your diet.

Just because something is good for us, consuming it in excessive quantities is not necessarily good for us either, except perhaps for kale. Even that could be a problem if you were eating it to the exclusion of other, just as important foods. A diet excessive even in foods that are good for us does not reflect a balanced, well-nourished life.

It's a good idea to keep a journal of the foods you try, noting any reactions you notice. Do you experience bloating or gas after eating them? Pay attention to your body and don't introduce more than one different food at a time.

It's equally important to understand there is not usually one answer or fix for anything and that includes chronic disease. Claims that eating or drinking a particular food or beverage, however packed with nutrients and "super" it may be, is *the* cure for what ails you should be treated with the proper amount of suspicion. A well-balanced nutrient dense selection of nature made foods is what you're looking for.

So here we go. First, you'll see a list of dishes and whether they are used for breakfast, lunch, dinner, snacks or desserts. Following that are the recipes themselves in alphabetical order. At the end, you'll see the section on combining dishes to produce delicious, nutritious dinners in minutes.

Meal Combinations
3 Hours – 14 Recipes – 21 Meals – 12 Snacks – 6 Desserts
17 Servings of Superfoods – 36 Servings of Vegetables
7 Days of Total Nutrition

	Breakfast	Lunch	Dinner	Snack	Dessert
Blueberry Chia Pudding	x			x	
Roasted Broccoli With Sesame Seeds	x	x	x	x	
Cauliflower Rice with Peas & sautéed Bok Choy	x	x	x	x	
Chicken or Bean Salad with Creamy Cashew Dressing		x	x	x	
Energy Balls	x			x	x
Kale Salad with Beans & Chopped herbs	x	x	x	x	
Kale Stir Fry		x	x	x	

Mint Chocolate Mousse				x	x
Mixed Salad with Roasted Fennel		x	x	x	
Mushroom Alfredo Sauce with Cauliflower Rice		x	x	x	
Fresh Fruit with Orange Cashew Cream				x	x
Roasted Root Vegetables with Creamy Dressing & herbs	x	x	x	x	
Sunshine Porridge	x			x	x
Super Green Smoothie	x			x	x

Adapted from "How To Make Meals Work" www.andreabeaman.com

Serving Sizes
1 Cup Raw Leafy Vegetables (about the size of a small fist)
½ Cup of other vegetables
1 Cup of Fruit
1 Medium Fruit or ¼ Cup Dried Fruit or berries

Recipes
Blueberry Chia Pudding
¼ Cup Chia Seeds
1½ Cups Coconut Milk
1 TSP Vanilla Extract
¼ Cup Blueberries - Fresh or frozen
½ to 1 TSP Maple Syrup or Honey

Prep Time: 10 Minutes   **Cook Time: 0**   **Makes 4 x ½ Pint Servings**

Directions

1. Place the chia seeds in a bowl, add the coconut milk and vanilla and mix until combined.
2. Let sit for 15 to 30 minutes to allow chia seeds to absorb the milk and start to gel.
3. Mix again and place in the refrigerator overnight.
4. Pour the blueberries into a mason jar; add the maple syrup or honey, then top with the chia pudding mixture.

For an added layer of flavor and crunch, sprinkle with chopped pumpkin or sunflower seeds.

Chia seeds are considered a superfood and provide sustained energy. They are a great substitute for high carb breakfasts and snacks.

Roasted Broccoli with Sesame Seeds

Prep Time: 60 Seconds   Cook Time: 10–15 Minutes Vegetable Servings: 8

Directions

1. Heat oven to 400 degrees.
2. Toss 2lbs broccoli in 2 - 3 TBSP coconut oil.
3. Place in an ovenproof dish, season with salt and pepper and bake for 20 minutes.
4. Remove from the oven, sprinkle with sesame seeds and serve.

Cashew Base

I have cashew base on hand pretty much all the time in my kitchen because its super easy to make and can be turned into so many things. It has little taste and takes on the flavors of whatever you add to it.

Prep Time: 2 Minutes   Cooking Time: 0 Minutes   Makes 4 Cups

Directions

1. Place 1 Cup of raw cashews in a Mason jar or dish, cover with water and soak overnight in the refrigerator or for a minimum of 6 hours to plump up the nuts.
2. Drain, rinse in cold water, then place in a blender with just enough water to cover the nuts.
3. Blend to a smooth consistency.
4. Store refrigerated for up to 7 days.

You can use cashew base as an alternative to cream and wherever you would use cream in sauces. It's very versatile and can be used in as many ways as your imagination will allow. Here are some of my favorites.

Dairy Free Ranch Dressing

1Cup Cashew Base
2 TBSP Flax or Hemp Seed Oil
1 Clove of garlic, minced
3 TBSP Chives
3 TBSP Parsley
1 TSP White Wine Vinegar
Salt and pepper to taste

Prep Time: 10 Minutes   **Cooking Time: 0 Minutes**   **Makes 1 ¼ Cups**

Directions

Place all the ingredients in a blender and combine until smooth and creamy.

Using lemon juice instead of white wine vinegar and different herbs can change the taste of this delicious dressing. Try using tarragon with chicken and root vegetable dishes, or mint for a cooling effect with spicy food.

www.mywholefoodlife.com

Alfredo Sauce
1 Small onion, diced
1 -2 Cloves garlic, chopped
1Cup Cashew Base
1 TBSP Lemon Juice
1 – 2Cups of vegetable or meat broth
Coconut Oil
Salt and pepper to taste

Prep Time: 10 Minutes   **Cooking Time: 15 Minutes**   **Makes 2 Servings**

Directions
1. Sauté the onion and garlic in coconut oil over medium heat until soft and translucent.
2. Add the cashew base, lemon juice and stock and reduce the heat, stirring constantly. The sauce thickens quickly so be ready with more stock if it gets too thick.
3. Season with salt and pepper and simmer for 5 to 10 minutes before serving.

Add some mushrooms when sautéing the onion and garlic and serve over vegetables for a delicious meal.

Orange Cashew Cream
1Cup Cashew Base
¼ TSP Vanilla Extract
½ TSP Grated Orange Rind
2 TSP Honey

Prep Time: 5 Minutes   **Cooking Time: 0**   **Makes 1Cup**

Directions

Mix all ingredients together and chill in the refrigerator.

This is a delicious dip for cut fruit and great as an afternoon snack or as a dessert.

www.wheatbelly.com

Basic Cauliflower Rice
1 Head of Cauliflower
2 TSPS Coconut Oil
1 TSP Sesame Oil (Optional)
½ Cup Finely Diced Yellow Onion
1 Clove of Garlic
½ Cup Water

Prep Time: 10 Minutes   **Cook Time: 12 Minutes**   **Vegetable Servings: 8 - 12**

Directions

1. Place the cauliflower florets in a food processor fitted with a grating attachment and process until grated into "rice grains." Alternatively, grate the cauliflower with a cheese grater.
2. Heat the oil in a large skillet or wok over a medium-high heat. Add the onion and garlic and sauté for 5 minutes.
3. Add the riced cauliflower and continue cooking for 5 to 7 minutes until the onions are translucent.
4. Add the water, cover and steam for 5 minutes until the cauliflower is cooked and the water is absorbed.

Danielle Walker, "Against All Grain"

Energy Balls

Of all the recipes, this is perhaps the most time consuming, taking about fifteen minutes of preparation and assembly. That said, one batch produces enough energy balls for five snacks, desserts or breakfasts and you can easily double the recipe for a week's worth of delicious fuel.

I also had to include this recipe because it was the first truly gluten, dairy and grain free food I had tasted and my body knew the difference immediately. It was because I ate these for three days, in place of wheat, gluten, cereals and pastas, that I became aware of the changes in my body. It took just three days to realize the stabbing, throbbing pain in my muscles had just about gone, that my joints were no longer constantly aching and my mind was starting to put those all important thoughts together in some kind of order at last!

½ Cup Unsweetened Shredded Coconut
¼ Cup Sunflower Seeds
4 Dates, Pits removed
2 TBSP Dried Cranberries
2 TBSP Coconut Oil
2 TBSP Raw Cacao Powder

Prep Time: 15 Minutes   **Cooking Time: 0**   **Makes about 10 x 1½ Balls**

Directions

1. Put the first three ingredients in a food processor and blend until finely chopped.
2. Melt the coconut oil, remove from the heat and add the raw cacao powder.
3. Mix the wet and dry ingredients, form into balls and place in the refrigerator to set. If the mixture is too sticky to form into balls, put it in the fridge for ten or fifteen minutes so it's easier to work with.

www.primallyinspired.com

Additions

You can add all kinds of dried fruit to this recipe in place of the cranberries, or none at all. I sometimes add a tablespoon of cinnamon and spirulina to my batches. The spirulina gives another layer of nutrition and fuel and the cinnamon tastes delicious. It is also a powerful antioxidant, helping my body rid itself of damaging free radicals produced by the process of living.

Don't be afraid to experiment and have fun with this recipe. There are never any failures, just some experiments that work and taste better than others and serendipity can produce some delicious "mistakes!"

Kale Salad
6 – 8 Cups Kale
3 - 4 TBSP Lemon Juice
1 Avocado
Salt and Pepper to taste

Prep Time: 2 Minutes   Cook Time: 0 Minutes   Vegetable Servings: 7-9

Directions

1. Place the raw, chopped and washed kale in a bowl.
2. Sprinkle with the lemon juice and let sit for thirty minutes so the juice can start to break down the kale fibers.
3. Cut up a large avocado and squish into the kale with your hands.
4. Season with sea salt and pepper.

Store in the refrigerator and use as a side dish, a snack or the base for a delicious salad. Add some chopped tomatoes and sprinkle with pumpkin seeds for an instant lunch.

Mint Chocolate Mousse

1 Ripe Avocado
1 Can Full Fat Coconut Milk
3 TBSP Raw Cacao Powder
2 - 3 TBSP Maple Syrup or Honey
1 TSP Vanilla Extract
½ TSP Mint Extract
Pinch of Salt
Shredded Coconut or Blueberries to Garnish

Prep Time: 5 Minutes   Cook Time: 0 Minutes   Makes 4 Servings

Directions

1. Scoop the avocado out of its skin.
2. Place in a blender with all the other ingredients except the garnish and pulse to mix.
3. Blend until well combined and creamy.
4. Pour into serving dishes and garnish with the shredded coconut or blueberries.
5. Refrigerate for an hour before serving.

Adapted from "The Immune System Recovery Plan" by Susan BLUM, M.D.
www.blumcenterforhealth.com

Roasted Root Vegetables
Prep Time: 5 Minutes   Cook Time: 20 Minutes
½ CUP Cooked Vegetables is 1 serving

Roasting any vegetable in coconut oil at high temperatures transforms it from the horrors of your childhood into what you'd imagine something from the Garden of Eden might taste like. That's a lot of poetic license I know, but honestly, this is one life tip you need to take at absolute face value.

Toss anything in coconut oil, put it in the oven for about twenty minutes at four hundred degrees and what comes out will astound you. I don't think there is any vegetable I haven't roasted and I have yet to find one that I didn't love.

Fennel bulbs, cut in half and roasted this way can be chopped and added to a salad, used as a garnish or drizzled with balsamic vinegar for an amazing side dish. Celeriac root, sweet potatoes, squash, Brussels sprouts, cabbage, carrots; how about a medley? Drizzle with creamy cashew ranch, sprinkle with chopped herbs and feel your energy reserves restored to overflowing.

Smoothies

Smoothies are a great way to get top quality nutrition into your body that can be instantly available as fuel. With a little knowledge, you can easily build your own smoothies. Start with a base of water, fruit juice, coconut water or nut milk. Next add vegetables, fruit and any protein or superfood you want.

Protein powders are processed foods even if the base ingredients are top quality, and cheaper, unprocessed alternatives are available that are just as nutritious. How about adding hemp or sesame seeds instead? Or how about some cashews or almonds, perhaps some flax or chia seeds, even half an avocado? Choose your protein source based on what your body needs, not what's on the ingredient list of even the best quality protein powder money can buy. They are no substitute for nature made and packaged foods.

I have included a recipe for my favorite smoothie below, but I often interchange ingredients, so again, don't be afraid to have fun. If there is a way to go "wrong" with smoothies, it's in using fruit juices that are very high in sugar as a base, then piling more fruit on top of that. Aim for a good balance with more vegetables than fruit. If you are adding fruit, it may be a good idea to use something other than fruit juice as your base.

You don't have to stick with kale either. Spinach, lettuce, chard and things like cucumber can add great flavor, as can different herbs.

Sue's Super Green Smoothie

2 Cups Water, Coconut Water or Unsweetened Coconut Milk
2 Good Handfuls of Kale
Generous Sprig of Parsley
Generous Sprig of Cilantro
1 Banana
½ to ¾ Cup Blueberries
2 TBSP Hemp Seeds, Sesame Seeds or Nut Butter
2 TSP Spirulina

Prep Time: 5 Minutes   **Serving Size: 2 x 16oz Servings**

Directions

Place all ingredients in a blender and put on "Chop" setting until combined. Switch to "Smoothie" setting until desired consistency, pour and enjoy!

This versatile recipe can be adapted to suit what you have on hand as well as the fruits that are in season. Packed full of powerful antioxidants, protein, fiber, healthy fats and amino acids that are instantly available to your cells, this delicious smoothie also contains important electrolytes and trace minerals. I feel my body come alive every time I drink this!

Sunshine Porridge

1 ½ Cups Coconut or other nut milk
½ Cup Pumpkin Seed Flour*
½ Cup Sunflower Seed Flour*
¼ Cup Hemp Seed Flour*
¼ Cup Chia Seeds*
2 TBSP Coconut Flour
½ TSP Cardamom
Generous Pinch Sea Salt
2 Eggs
1½ TBSP Maple Syrup or Honey

1 TSP Vanilla
2 TBSP Coconut Butter or Coconut Oil
½ to 1 CUP chopped strawberries, or other fruit

Prep Time: 10 minutes   Cook Time: 10 Minutes   Servings: 4

Directions

1. Whisk the dry ingredients together and set aside.
2. Whisk wet ingredients together and slowly add to dry mixture.
3. Place in a small saucepan and bring to a boil over medium heat, stirring constantly. Add the coconut oil or coconut butter and reduce heat to medium-low and stir about 3 minutes until thick and creamy.
4. Top with fruit and chopped nuts.

* Use a coffee or spice grinder to grind pumpkin, sunflower, chia and hemp seeds.
Adapted from http://freecoconutrecipes.com/grain-free-strawberries-n-cream-porridge/

Dinner Combinations
Mix and Match Meals

Though there are many more recipes at the From Couch To Life! website, I want to show you how the recipes above can be combined to provide a multitude of dishes. With a few additions, you'll be able to give yourself the top quality nutrition you need without using a ton of time and energy doing it.

Additions

Adding a high quality protein from a vegetable or animal source, some great salad items like chopped tomatoes, cucumbers and grated carrot, a few chopped herbs as a garnish and you have convenient total nutrition that tastes delicious.

For dinner, how about cauliflower rice served on a bed of mixed salad greens, topped with roasted root vegetables, drizzled with cashew dressing and sprinkled with sesame seeds? A serving of mint chocolate avocado mousse would finish off the meal nicely, if you had any room left!

Here are some more of my favorites.

Kale Stir Fry

Sauté kale in coconut oil with two cloves of garlic, add a handful of cherry tomatoes and season with salt and pepper. Cook for five to ten minutes, transfer to your plate, add half a sliced avocado, cover with cashew Ranch dressing, sprinkle with chopped herbs and devour!

Mixed Salad with Roasted Fennel

Start with a bed of greens, add grated carrot, maybe some chopped tomatoes, top with roasted fennel and dress with balsamic vinegar and olive oil.

Chicken and Broccoli

If you eat meat, buying a whole chicken that has already been cooked can save a ton of time. Make sure you buy humanely raised, organic pastured chicken for top nutrition free of hormones and antibiotics.

Beans, already cooked, are a great alternative to animal protein.

Chicken or Bean Salad with Creamy Ranch Dressing

Now you have the idea, the following suggestions are pretty self explanatory. When it comes to salads, add whatever you like. Tomatoes, cucumber and grated carrot are my favorites, and adding chopped basil, cilantro, tarragon and mint to your salad can complement the dish perfectly.

Roasted vegetable medley with pumpkin seeds and dressing

Serve these over a bed of mixed salad greens. The heat from the vegetable will wilt the greens and a few slices of avocado would add a great finishing touch.

Cauliflower rice with Peas and roasted Bok Choy

Add frozen peas and roasted Bok Choy to a batch of basic cauliflower rice.

Kale Salad with chicken or beans and fresh chopped herbs

If you were to make all these recipes, you would have spent about three hours in the kitchen and produced twenty-one meals, twelve snacks and six desserts. In addition, you'll have consumed more than six pounds of vegetables and two pounds of fruit. Fuel and medicine to power the life you now have back!

Food Lists

- **Big 8 Top Allergy Foods and Food Intolerances**
- **Detox Foods**
- **Drinks**
- **Fats and Oils**
- **Superfoods**
- **Substitutions for Top Allergy Foods**
  Egg Substitutes
  Flours
  Gluten Substitutes
  Non-Dairy Milk
  Sugar Substitutions
  Thickening Agents (non animal and gluten)
  Yeast Free Baking and Dairy and Nut Free Butters

Big 8 Top Allergy Foods

The FDA requires all food manufacturers to list any ingredient on the top eight food allergens lists on product labels and you may be surprised at what's on this list. Add to that the increasing number of people with food intolerances, and it may not be such a surprise that so many people experience an improvement in their symptoms when they make diet and lifestyle changes.

Take a look at some of the food in your kitchen and see how many labels list the following ingredients and how many of these things you eat on a regular basis.

- Milk
- Eggs
- Peanuts
- Tree nuts (such as almond, cashews, walnuts)
- Fish (such as bass, cod, flounder)
- Shellfish (such as crab, lobster, shrimp)
- Soy
- Wheat

Food Intolerances

- Gluten
- Lactose[9]

Great Detox Foods

Though many people look at detox as a "sometimes," thing, usually when things start to go awry, eating whole foods ensures you always have what you need to get rid of what your body doesn't want or need.

Our bodies are continually detoxing themselves, through the obvious channels, for which we use our bathrooms, as well as the not so obvious, our

---

9   http://www.fda.gov/Food/ResourcesForYou/Consumers/ucm079311.htm

sweat and our lungs. The idea that we have to go on a special diet to get rid of the nasty build up of toxins we accumulate as a part of everyday living, doesn't help us understand how we can support this already efficient and inbuilt systems with its task.

Many, many foods have the ability to assist your body in detoxing, but below is a selection of some of the superstars. Cruciferous vegetables (meaning those of the cabbage family), like broccoli, kale and of, course, cabbage, help increase the enzymes in the body that help us detox. Herbs contain substances called chelators that attach themselves to heavy metals and sulfur rich foods like onions, garlic and eggs help eliminate them from the body. Pectin in fruit helps eliminate metals as well as drug residues.

If all these delicious foods make it into your diet on a regular basis, you can be sure that as soon as your ever vigilant body spots an intruder, it can unleash the full power of say parsley and cauliflower chemicals and the toxin is history!

Artichokes contain the antioxidant, silymarin that helps the liver process toxins, and cynarin that helps it break down fatty acids. Packed with fiber, protein, magnesium, folate and potassium, it is way more than a detox food.

Asparagus helps with liver drainage, is a powerful anti-inflammatory and is considered an anti ageing food.

Basil has antibacterial properties and antioxidants that protect the liver.

Beets are chock full of magnesium, iron, zinc and calcium that help flush out toxins.

Brazil Nuts are high in selenium, a key element in metabolism and an essential element that makes body processes work properly. It's great at removing mercury from the body, it enhances the action of antioxidants and just two Brazil nuts a day should be all you need.

Broccoli. What can't I say about this beautiful flowering head of a vegetable? Is there *anything* it can't do? Well yes, as we learned in the mind/body connection, it does not have the power to save you from a life of loneliness and despair, but despite this shortcoming, it can do pretty much everything else. Working with liver enzymes, it helps turn those noxious toxins into something the body can get rid of.

Cabbage, one of the cruciferous vegetables, increases the enzymes you need to detox and helps clean the liver in the process.

Cilantro is excellent at removing heavy metals like cadmium, aluminum, mercury and uranium that often lodge in the bones and nervous system.

Garlic is high in vitamin C, a great support to the immune system and liver.

Grapefruit floods the body with dense nutrition that fires up the liver and helps burn fat. Its effects on weight loss are well documented, as are its effect on some heart medications, so check with your doctor before you eat this fruit.

Onions suck up arsenic, lead, cadmium and mercury while helping the liver get rid of toxins.

Parsley is full of beta-carotene and vitamins A, C and K, which help to protect the kidneys and bladder. A great chelator, it is especially good at removing mercury.

Pineapple cleanses the colon and its high enzyme content, especially of bromelain, help the intestines break down waste.

Sesame Seeds protect the liver from alcohol and other toxins.

www.bembu.com/data-foods

Drinks

Though water is so essential to life, so many live lives of quiet dehydration. Tiredness, headaches, hunger and cravings are often treated with sugar and other foods in the mistaken belief that lack of energy is the cause of symptoms. Though many find it immensely boring to drink it and some say they gag on the stuff, adding some of the following to water can make it easier to stay well hydrated.

Flavored Water

Citrus fruits like lemon, lime and orange are delicious. Try adding a slice or two to your glass.

Herbs like mint and basil make a very refreshing addition to water. Crush the leaves a little to release even more flavor and some of their powerful health benefits.

Essential Oils, food grade of course, can be a wonderful addition. Try cinnamon or clove for a great boost and something completely different. Be careful with essential oils, they are potent and can cause symptoms similar to pollen allergies. Digestive issues can also occur, so proceed with caution and don't be tempted to use more than is advised by the manufacturer.

Milk Based Drinks

Hot Chocolate

Two or three cups of warmed, unsweetened coconut milk, a tablespoon of raw cacao powder, a half teaspoon of cardamom, a sprinkle of nutmeg and a kiss of honey will reenergize you and transport you half way round the world with its intoxicating blend of spices.

Hemp Milk is packed with protein and is another great drink to use as an afternoon pick me up. I add nutmeg and a little coconut oil for added energy and can work for hours before I feel the need to refuel.

Other Drinks

Coconut Water is full of important electrolytes so it can be particularly good at rehydrating you. It's a great alternative to commercial sports drinks that are often loaded with added sugars, flavorings and dyes.

Kombucha is a slightly fizzy drink made by fermenting tea using beneficial bacteria and yeast and is full of probiotics that help support the digestive system contributing to overall health.

Teas, from black to green, made from leaves, flowers, herbs or roots, either hot or cold, are packed with important nutrients and protective elements. Many of you may be familiar with the powerful antioxidants in green tea, but many others teas can be a surprising source of important minerals.

Rooibos, from South Africa, is one such tea. It is caffeine free, high in vitamin C, and a surprising source of calcium and magnesium. It's another one of my favorite afternoon "pick me ups," and the high levels of vitamin C can be very helpful in treating certain skin conditions, like acne.

Echinacea is also packed with vitamin C and soothing to the throat. Chai tea, with its intoxicating aroma and warm spices makes drinking it way more than a hydrating experience. Jasmine, perhaps with a delicate dried rose bud will refresh you and help restore balance.

Another Note of Caution

Some health conditions can be affected by certain foods, however whole and organic they may be. Essential oils have powerful anti bacterial, anti fungal and anti viral properties and I can attest to the fact that using them internally is not always a good idea. In some cases, they can also interfere with the proper function of medications, so the "Necessary Note of Caution," bears repeating here. Check with your doctor or health care provider before using them and making changes in your diet.

Fats and Oils[10]

Here's the lowdown on fat, what each one is, what they do in the body and what happens when we don't have enough or too much of the wrong ones. Following that is a list of substitutions for butter in cooking and finally, some fat free options.

- Fats are very important for many things, but chiefly for the integrity of cell membranes (omega 6's), and the functioning of the brain, (omega 3's), the brain being more than sixty percent fat.
- The most health promoting fats are monounsaturated and polyunsaturated fats.
- Omega 6's are generally pro-inflammatory; a good thing that protects against infections and promotes healing.
- Omega 3's are generally anti-inflammatory and equally important. Among other things, they turn off the inflammatory response when it's no longer needed.
- An incorrect balance of omega 3's and 6's keeps the pre-inflammatory switch on, leading to chronic disease.
- Too little fat in the diet can lead to hormone abnormalities, cardiovascular disease and decreased immune and brain function.
- Too much butter and animal fat in the diet can lead to arteriosclerosis and heart disease.

---

10 Heart Disease and Diet http://www.nlm.nih.gov/medlineplus/ency/article/002436.htm
http://www.hsph.harvard.edu/nutritionsource/what-should-you-eat/fats-and-cholesterol/

Main Fat Groups

Saturated	Monounsaturated	Polyunsaturated
Coconut*, Avocado, Palm	Olive, Sunflower	Safflower, Sesame, Soybean, Flaxseed, Peanut Butter
Ghee is pure butter fat Contains no casein or lactose		The omega fats 3, 6 and 9
Solid at room temperature	Liquid at room temp Become solid when chilled	Liquid at room temp Remains liquid when chilled
Potentially increased risk of heart disease Generally recommended to limit consumption of butter.	Raise good HDL and lower LDL	Raises good HDL and lower LDL

* Solid up to 76 degrees when it becomes a liquid. Considered a saturated fat, it consists of short and medium chain fatty acids, known as triglycerides. They break down easily without the need for pancreatic enzymes or bile, the nutrients going straight to the liver. Rather than being stored as fat, they boost energy, the metabolism and the immune system.

Coconut oil makes food taste delicious. Though it doesn't have much taste itself, it does something incredible to just about anything cooked with it. It also has a high smoking point, making it idea for stir-fries and roasting vegetables in the oven at 400 degrees.

Superfoods
Nutrient dense anti oxidant rich and low calorie

Superfoods are nutrient dense, low calorie foods full of protein, fiber phytochemicals and antioxidants that provide endurance, fuel and medicine. A smoothie of superfoods is the ultimate body experience!

Top 10 Superfoods

1. Proteins – Spirulina, Hemp, a complete protein and Quinoa that has the highest protein content of any grain
2. Greens – Kale, Broccoli, Brussels sprouts, Collard Greens or anything green!
3. Fresh fruit, especially Apples, Bananas, Berries
4. Nuts and nut butters
5. Seeds, especially Flax, Sunflower, Pumpkin and Chia
6. Coconut oil, flesh and water are very high in fiber, vitamins, amino acids and protein
7. Raw cacao provides instant energy, is high in magnesium and raises endorphin and serotonin levels. It boosts brain power and helps energize the muscles
8. Seaweed, rich in minerals not found on land
9. Green and herbal Teas
10. Exotic Superfoods, like Maca, Goji and Acai Berries

Do you notice something about this list? It's actually a list of whole foods Mother Nature makes, in all the different places of the world. In South America, she makes the Gogi Berry, in England, the strawberry, in America, the blueberry. There are tons of others, many more exotic, hailing from all parts of the world. In truth every country and continent has its very own superfoods.

This isn't really a top ten list. They are so packed with goodness; they could all be at number one. Consume anything from this list on a regular basis and you'll see your energy levels soar.

They are nature made foods that are readily available and packed with nutrition.

Substitutions for the Big 8 Allergy Foods

Egg Substitutes
**Eggs add moisture and act as binding and leavening agents in baking.
Use any of the following to substitute for 1 Egg**

1 TBSP Tapioca 3 TBSP Water	Cakes, Cookies (Increase leavening agent e.g. baking soda, by ¼ TSP)
2 TBSP Potato Starch 3 TBSP Water	Cakes, Cookies
2 TBSP Arrowroot 3 TBSP Water	Cakes, Cookies
1 TBSP Flaxseed Meal* ½ TSP Baking Powder 3 TBSP Water	Breads. Can make the product gummy in the center, especially if using Rice Flour in the recipe
1 TBSP Chia Seeds ⅛ TSP Baking Powder 3 TBSP Water	Breads. Can make the product gummy in the center, especially if using Rice Flour
⅓ Cup Apple Sauce	Cakes and Brownies
½ Mashed Banana or ¼ Cup ¼ TSP Baking Powder	Cakes and Brownies
3 TBSP Pureed Fruit	Cakes and Brownies
1 TSP Baking Soda 1 TBSP Vinegar or Lemon Juice	

¼ Cup Vegetable Oil

Egg White Substitute   1 TBSP Agar 1 TBSP Water
                                        Whip, chill, and then whip again

* Some people have a hard time digesting flaxseeds and flaxseed meal, so watch for digestive distress from gas and bloating.

www.glutenfreegoddess.com/2008/12/baking-cooking-substitutions-
for-gluten.htm

Oil Substitutions in Recipes

In baking, butter is used to add rich flavor and a spongy texture. It helps baked goods rise evenly, and adds density and sweetness.

Coconut Oil	1:1 Ratio	Silky texture	Biscuits. Use solid as shortening
		Mild taste	Thickens as butter does
Olive Oil	1:1 Ratio		Breads, muffins and cakes that use herbs, citrus and strong flavors like pumpkin
Other Oils		1-2 TBSP less to start	

www.veganbaking.com

Naturally Fat Free Options in Baking

Applesauce is great in muffins, cookies, cakes and recipes that use fruit, nuts, ginger and cardamom. Its tangy quality makes it a challenge when pared with chocolate. Canned pumpkin, sweet potato cooked and mashed and organic baby foods also add body and moisture without fat.

Tip: Pair strong fruit flavors with other strong flavors in recipes, like cinnamon, nutmeg, molasses and ginger.

Vegan Baking Substitution Guide at www.veganbaking.com

Gluten Substitutes

Gluten is the "glue" that helps stick baked goods together. Cooking without it produces a crumbly, more fragile result. Here is a list of alternatives:

	Alternatives	
Guar Gum	Legume Based	Avoid if sensitive to beans, soy or lentils
Xanthum Gum	Cellulose	Avoid if sensitive to corn
1 TBSP Potato Starch		Has binding ability, especially when whisked with warm liquid
Tapioca Starch		

Arrowroot
Extra Egg White

1 -2 TBSP Honey or Agave	Adds moisture and binding
1 TBSP Flaxseed Gel	Adds great texture and fiber.
(1 TBSP Flaxseed meal: 3 TBSP Water)	Doesn't bind as well
½ Cup Fruit Jam	Helps bind and adds moisture. Use in muffins and quick breads

Gluten Free Flours
Light, Starchy Flours – Delicate, melt in your mouth, baked goods

Sweet Rice*	Very sticky. Dissolves in the mouth. Use ¼ Cup max. per recipe. Mostly interchangeable with Tapioca Flour

Tapioca	Browns well. A little tough. Mix with Potato starch or Arrowroot to soften
Cornstarch	Light and springy texture. Combine with Arrowroot for softness and a golden crust
Potato Starch	Breads, Muffins, Cakes Do not use Potato Flour that is heavy, gooey and best used to thicken gravies

Medium Flours – Like All Purpose Flour

Sorghum aka Jowar	
Gluten Free Oat Flour	Closest to Sorghum
Brown Rice *	A better choice for baking but can be gummy so add fiber and starch

* Due to the high, naturally occurring arsenic content of rice, using it in large quantities is not advisable.

Heavy flours – Like Whole Wheat
Dense, darker, less rise

Quinoa	
Buckwheat	Member of rhubarb family, aka Kasha.
Millet	
Cornmeal	Tender, sweet, slightly grainy texture, aka polenta
Almond Flour	Substitute 1:1 for sunflower* and/or pumpkin seed flour
Bean / Legume	Can have metallic taste and be hard to digest. Soy and chickpea flour aka garbanzo are starchier. Use small amounts to minimize blood sugar rise. Try ½ Cup

Nut Free Flours

Coconut	Fiber rich and highly absorbent. Add more liquid or fat Let sit to gauge consistency Use as a secondary flour	
Flaxseed or almond		
Sesame Seed	Choose lighter varieties	
Pumpkin Seed Meal	Slightly spicy flavor. Great pared with the warm spices of cinnamon, nutmeg and cardamom	Muffins Breads
Hemp	Heavy, dense and very moist	Gives great buttery flavor
Sunflower Seed	Light to medium flour. Great when blended with hemp and pumpkin seed meal	Scones

* Baking soda reacts with the chlorogenic acid found in sunflower seeds to turn baked goods green, fabulous for St. Patrick's Day. For every other day of the year, halving the baking soda or keeping the sunflower seed flour content to ¼ cup or less of the flour mixture in a recipe should minimize or cancel this effect. I have also substituted baking powder for baking soda with success in many recipes.

Tips for Successful Baking and Substitutions
- The best blends are a mixture of medium and heavy flours, plus a starch
- Higher protein flours produce a more tender texture
- Substitute flour by weight
- Substitute light for light, medium for medium and heavy for heavy

- Adjust moisture levels when substituting flours
- Batters are stiffer than wheat flours at first, then stretch, then get sticky
- Starches lighten, bind and tenderize
- Add ¼ Cup Flaxseed meal to increase fiber content
- If gummy or sinking in the middle, increase oven temperature 25 – 50 degrees or add more fiber. (See above)

www.glutenfreegoddess.com

Non-Dairy Milk

Almond Milk	Creamy, slightly nutty	Good all round milk
Cashew Milk	Smooth, creamy, slightly nutty, sweet and rich. Comparable to whole milk	Cooking, desserts, whipped vegetables, making cream
Coconut Milk	Smooth, silky, not strong Comparable to semi skimmed / reduced fat milk	Sauces, soups, curries, cereals, hot drinks, smoothies, whipped vegetables
Hazelnut Milk	Light, rich nutty flavor Delicious in coffee	Drinks and light desserts. Not suitable for cooking and baking
Hemp Milk	Rich, Creamy, strong flavor Not so good in hot drinks*	Creamy sauces, especially savory dishes, smoothies, ice cream, soups
Oat Milk	Creamy and naturally sweet	Good for cooking. A little heavy for baking

| Rice Milk | Thin, watery consistency Similar consistency to skimmed milk | Great on cereal and in cooking. Too light and watery for hot drinks |

www.veganbandit.com

* Hemp milk may not taste so good *in* drinks, but as an afternoon pick me up, you can't beat a warm mug of hemp milk, lightly sweetened with honey and sprinkled with freshly ground nutmeg. Packed with protein, fats and antioxidants, it will keep you going into the early evening.

Sugar Substitutions – 1 Cup White Sugar
Tips: Use less liquid sweetener than sugar.
Overall volume may be less. Adjust pan size.

Agave Nectar	⅔ Cup	Lower oven by 25 degrees
Barley Malt	1 – 1 ½ Cups	
Birch Syrup (Xylitol)	1 Cup	Doesn't work well in bread or hard candy
Brown Rice Syrup	1 – 1 ½ Cups	Good for hard or crunchy baked goods
Coconut Crystals	1 Cup	
Date Sugar	⅔ Cup	Burns easily
Erythritol	1 – ¼ Cups	
Honey	Reduce by ¼ Cup	If no liquid, add 3 TBSP flour for each ½ Cup honey
Maple Syrup	Reduce by 3 TBSP	Add ¼ TSP Baking soda
Maple Sugar	½ - ⅓ Cup	Add ⅛ TSP Baking Soda
Molasses	1 – 1 ⅓ Cups	
Rapidura	1 Cup	Less refined cane sugar
Stevia	Add ⅛ Cup	Experiment for right ratio
Sucanat	1 Cup	Add ¼ TSP Baking Soda

Turbinado	1 Cup	Less refined cane sugar
Vegetable Glycerin	4 TBSP	

Thickening Agents

Agar Agar	1 TBSP : 4 TBSP Water	Vegetable gelatin	
Arrowroot	1:1 with Cold Water	Stir over low heat	Gravy and Sauces
Cashew Base	1 Cup Cashews 1 – 1 ½ Cups Water	Rich, creamy, thickens quickly. Add plenty of liquid when cooking	Sauces, soups, stews, salad dressings, cream
Cauliflower Mash			
Cornstarch		Doesn't freeze well Doesn't reheat well Gives glossy look	Gravy and sauces
Egg Yolks			Sauces, Soup bases, mayonnaise
Gelatin	1 TBSP Gelatin 3 TBSP Warm water	Animal based	Desserts
Kudzu, Aka Kuzu	1 TBSP Kudzu 2 TBSP Cold water to 1 Cup liquid		Sauces, pie fillings, desserts, gravy, soups
Potato	Mashed		
Potato Starch	Kosher	Grain free option Gets lumpy, stir often	Gravy and sauces
Potato Flour		Thickens and clumps easily	

| Sweet Rice Flour Sorghum | 1:1 with water | Sticky | Roux based sauces |
| Tapioca Starch aka Manioc, Yucca, Cassava | 1:1 with water | Thickens quickly Add at end of cooking | |

www.glutenfreegoddess.com

Yeast Free Baking

What could you possibly use in recipe in place of yeast, if you have to avoid it?

| 1 TSP Baking Soda 1 TSP Lemon Juice or 1 TSP Apple Cider Vinegar | Forms carbon dioxide bubbles immediately |
| Baking Powder | Forms carbon dioxide bubbles when it reaches a certain temperature |

www.glutenfreegoddess.com

Dairy and Nut Free Butters

Sunflower Seed Butter, aka Sun Butter
Pumpkin Seed Butter
Cashew Butter
Sesame Seed butter, also known as tahini
Hemp Butter

Resources

sue@fromcouch2life.com

www.fromcouchtolife.com

Against All Grain	www.againstallgrain.com
Biology of Belief	https://biologyofbelief.wordpress.com
Blum Center for Heath	www.blumcenterforhealth.com
Clean Plates - Organic, sustainable and non-GMO Restaurant list	www.cleanplates.com
Chronic Fatigue Syndrome Knowledge Center	www.cfsknowledecenter.com
Eat To Live – Dr. Fuhrman	www.drfuhrman.com
Environmental Working Group – EWG	
Clean 15 and Dirty Dozen	www.ewg.org/foodnews
Cosmetics Database	www.ewg.org/skindeep
Food Allergies - The "Big 8"	www.foodallergy.org
Gluten Free Goddess	www.glutenfreegoddess.blogspot.com
My Whole food Life	www.mywholefoodlife.com
Institute for Integrative Nutrition®	http://www.integrativenutrition.com
Oh My Veggies	www.ohmyveggies.com
Primally Inspired	www.primallyinspired.com
Rotary International	www.rotary.org
Seafood Watch	www.seafoodwatch.org
Vegan Bandit	www.veganbandit.net
World's Healthiest Foods	www.whfoods.com
Wheat Belly	www.wheatbelly.com

Index